Prefix
MTW

0009884

KT-558-008

Study Guide to Accompany

Essentials of
Nursing Research

METHODS, APPRAISAL, AND UTILIZATION

SIXTH EDITION

The Library, Ed & Trg Centre   KTW
Tunbridge Wells Hospital
Tonbridge Rd, PEMBURY
Kent TN2 4QJ
01892 635884 and 635489

Books must be returned/renewed by the last date shown

31st Aug.   0 8 APR 2021

3 0 AUG 2006

1 3 OCT 2006   - 4 SEP 2009

2 3 OCT 2006   1 3 APR 2010

6 AUG 2007   2 8 AUG 2012   DISCARDED

1 3 MAR 2008

8 April 08   2 0 DEC 2012

5 JAN 2009   1 2 FEB 2015

- 5 JAN 2016

2 6 SEP 2017

Study Guide to Accompany

Essentials of Nursing Research

METHODS, APPRAISAL, AND UTILIZATION

SIXTH EDITION

Denise F. Polit, PhD
President
Humanalysis, Inc.
Saratoga Springs, New York

Cheryl Tatano Beck, DNSc, CNM, FAAN
Professor
University of Connecticut, School of Nursing
Storrs, Connecticut

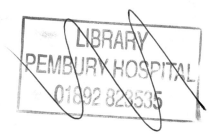
LIBRARY
PEMBURY HOSPITAL
01892 823535

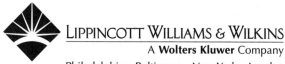

LIPPINCOTT WILLIAMS & WILKINS
A **Wolters Kluwer** Company
Philadelphia • Baltimore • New York • London
Buenos Aires • Hong Kong • Sydney • Tokyo

Ancillary Editor: *Doris S. Wray*
Senior Managing Editor, Production: *Erika Kors*
Senior Production Manager: *Helen Ewan*
Design Coordinator: *Brett MacNaughton*
Manufacturing Manager: *William Alberti*

Sixth Edition

Copyright © 2006 Lippincott Williams & Wilkins. Copyright © 2001 Lippincott Williams & Wilkins. Copyright © 1997 by Lippincott-Raven Publishers. Copyright © 1993, by J.B. Lippincott Company. Copyright © 1989, by J.B. Lippincott Company. Copyright © 1985, by J.B. Lippincott Company. All rights reserved. This book is protected by copyright. No part of it may be reproduced, stored in a retrieval system, or transmitted, in any form or by any means—electronic, mechanical, photocopy, recording, or otherwise—without the prior written permission of the publisher. Printed in the United States of America. For information write Lippincott Williams & Wilkins, 530 Walnut St., Philadelphia, PA 19106.

Materials appearing in this book prepared by individuals as part of their official duties as U.S. Government employees are not covered by the above-mentioned copyright.

10 9 8 7 6 5 4 3 2 1

ISBN: 0-7817-7679-1

Care has been taken to confirm the accuracy of the information presented and to describe generally accepted practices. However, the authors, editors, and publisher are not responsible for errors or omissions or for any consequences from application of the information in this book and make no warranty, express or implied, with respect to the contents of the publication.

The authors, editors and publisher have exerted every effort to ensure that drug selection and dosage set forth in this text are in accordance with current recommendations and practice at the time of publication. However, in view of ongoing research, changes in government regulations, and the constant flow of information relating to drug therapy and drug reactions, the reader is urged to check the package insert for each drug for any change in indications and dosage and for added warnings and precautions. This is particularly important when the recommended agent is a new or infrequently employed drug.

Some drugs and medical devices presented in this publication have Food and Drug Administration (FDA) clearance for limited use in restricted research settings. It is the responsibility of the health care provider to ascertain the FDA status of each drug or device planned for use in their clinical practice.

Preface

This Study Guide has been prepared to complement the sixth edition of *Essentials of Nursing Research: Methods, Appraisal, and Utilization.* As was true for the textbook, this Study Guide retains many features that have made it a useful learning tool in the past, but we have introduced numerous innovations designed to further bridge the gap between the passive reading of complex and abstract materials and the active development of skills needed to critique studies and use their findings in practice.

The guide provides you with opportunities to reinforce the acquisition of basic research skills through systematic learning exercises—some of which are designed to be "fun." For example, in this edition we have included crossword puzzles in every chapter, using key new terms that were introduced in the textbook. Another important new feature is that the appendices include seven research reports in their entirety (including one meta-analysis and one metasynthesis), and there are powerful activities in each chapter (the Application Exercises) geared around these studies.

The Study Guide consists of eighteen chapters—one chapter corresponding to every chapter in the textbook. Each of the eighteen chapters (with a few exceptions) consists of four sections:

- *Matching Exercises.* Terms and concepts presented in the textbook are reinforced by having you perform a matching routine that often involves matching the concrete (e.g., actual hypotheses) with the abstract (e.g., type of hypotheses).
- *Completion Exercises.* Sentences are presented in which you must fill in a missing word or phrase corresponding to important ideas presented in the textbook.
- *Study Questions.* Each chapter contains two to five short individual exercises relevant to the materials in the textbook, including the completion of a crossword puzzle.
- *Application Exercises.* These exercises are geared specifically to helping you to read, comprehend, and critique nursing research studies. In each chapter, the application exercises focus on two of the studies in the appendices—typically one qualitative and one quantitative study. For each study, there are two sets of questions—*Questions of Fact* and *Questions for Discussion.* The Questions of Fact will help you to read the report and find specific types of information related to the content covered in the textbook. For these questions, there are "right" and "wrong" answers. For example, a question might ask: How many people participated in this study? The Questions for Discussion, by contrast, require an assessment of the merits of various features of the study. For example, a question might ask: Were there *enough* people participating in this study? The second set of questions can be the basis for classroom discussions.

We hope that you will find these activities rewarding, enjoyable, and useful in your effort to develop skills for evidence-based nursing practice.

Copyright © 2006. Lippincott Williams & Wilkins. *Study Guide to Accompany Essentials of Nursing Research,* by Denise F. Polit and Cheryl Tatano Beck.

Contents

Copyright © 2006. Lippincott Williams & Wilkins. *Study Guide to Accompany Essentials of Nursing Research*, by Denise F. Polit and Cheryl Tatano Beck.

PART 1

Overview of Nursing Research

CHAPTER 1

Exploring Nursing Research

■ A. Matching Exercises

Match each statement in Set B with one of the paradigms in Set A. Indicate the letter corresponding to your response next to each item in Set B.

SET A

a. Positivist/postpositivist paradigm

b. Naturalist paradigm

c. Neither paradigm

d. Both paradigms

SET B   **RESPONSES**

1. Assumes that reality exists and that it can be objectively studied and known   _____

2. Subjectivity in inquiries is considered inevitable and desirable.   _____

3. Inquiries rely on external, empirical evidence collected through human senses.   _____

4. Assumes reality is a construction and that many constructions are possible   _____

5. Method of inquiry relies primarily on collecting and analyzing quantitative information.   _____

6. Method of inquiry relies primarily on collecting and analyzing narrative, qualitative information.   _____

7. Provides an overarching framework for inquiries undertaken by nurse researchers   _____

8. Inquiries give rise to emerging interpretations that are grounded in people's experiences.   _____

9. Inquiries are not constrained by ethical issues.   _____

10. Inquiries focus on discrete, specific concepts while attempting to control others.   _____

Copyright © 2006. Lippincott Williams & Wilkins. *Study Guide to Accompany Essentials of Nursing Research*, by Denise F. Polit and Cheryl Tatano Beck.

■ B. Completion Exercises

Write the words or phrases that correctly complete the sentences below.

1. Research in nursing began with _____.

2. During the early years, most nursing studies focused on _____
_____.

3. The entity that was established in 1993 to promote and financially support nursing research in the United States is _____.

4. The future direction of nursing research is likely to involve a continuing focus on
_____.

5. The most ingrained source of evidence, and the one that is the most difficult to challenge, is _____.

6. The paradigm that views reality as multiply constructed is the _____
_____ paradigm.

7. The "scientific method" has as its philosophical underpinnings a school of thought known as _____.

8. Evidence that is rooted in objective reality and gathered through the human senses is known as _____ evidence.

9. The assumption that all phenomena have antecedent causes is called _____
_____.

10. Because traditional scientific research is not concerned with isolated or unique phenomena, a major goal is _____
_____ beyond those involved in the study.

11. Researchers who reject the classical model of scientific inquiry criticize it for being overly _____.

12. The type of research that involves the systematic collection and analysis of controlled, numerical information is known as _____.

13. The type of research that involves the systematic collection and analysis of subjective, narrative materials is known as _____.

14. A specific aim of some qualitative research that asks "What is the name of this phenomenon?" is referred to as _____.

Copyright © 2006. Lippincott Williams & Wilkins. *Study Guide to Accompany Essentials of Nursing Research*, by Denise F. Polit and Cheryl Tatano Beck.

■ C. Study Questions

1. Complete the crossword puzzle at the end of the chapter, which uses terms and concepts presented in Chapter 1. (Puzzles may be removed for easier viewing.)

2. Why is it important for nurses who will never conduct their own research to understand research methods?

   _____

   _____

   _____

   _____

   _____

3. What are some potential consequences to the nursing profession if nurses stopped conducting their own research?

   _____

   _____

   _____

   _____

   _____

4. Below are descriptions of several research problems. Indicate whether you think the problem is best suited to a qualitative or quantitative approach, and explain your rationale.

   a. What is the decision-making process of AIDS patients seeking treatment?

      _____

      _____

   b. What effect does room temperature have on the colonization rate of bacteria in urinary catheters?

      _____

      _____

   c. What are sources of stress among nursing home residents?

      _____

      _____

Copyright © 2006. Lippincott Williams & Wilkins. *Study Guide to Accompany Essentials of Nursing Research*, by Denise F. Polit and Cheryl Tatano Beck.

d. Does therapeutic touch affect the vital signs of hospitalized patients?

_____

_____

e. What is the meaning of *hope* among Stage IV cancer patients?

_____

_____

f. What are the effects of prenatal instruction on the labor and delivery outcomes of pregnant women?

_____

_____

g. What are the health care needs of the homeless, and what barriers do they face in having those needs met?

_____

_____

5. What are some of the limitations of quantitative research? What are some of the limitations of qualitative research? Which approach seems best suited to address problems in which you might be interested? Why is that?

_____

_____

_____

_____

_____

■ D. Application Exercises

1. Read the abstract and introduction to the report by Gibbins and her colleagues ("Procedural Pain") in Appendix A. Then answer the following questions:

QUESTIONS OF FACT

a. Is this report an example of "disciplined research"?

_____

_____

Copyright © 2006. Lippincott Williams & Wilkins. *Study Guide to Accompany Essentials of Nursing Research*, by Denise F. Polit and Cheryl Tatano Beck.

b. Is this a qualitative or quantitative study?

_____

_____

c. What is the underlying paradigm of the study?

_____

_____

d. Does the study involve the collection of empirical evidence?

_____

_____

e. Is the purpose of this study identification, description, exploration, explanation, and/or prediction and control?

_____

_____

f. Is this study applied or basic research?

_____

_____

QUESTIONS FOR DISCUSSION

a. How relevant is this study to the actual practice of nursing?

_____

_____

b. Could this study have been conducted as _either_ a quantitative or qualitative study? Why or why not?

_____

_____

2. Read the abstract and introduction to the report by Rew ("Homeless Youth") in Appendix B. Then answer the following questions:

QUESTIONS OF FACT

a. Is this report an example of "disciplined research"?

_____

_____

Copyright © 2006. Lippincott Williams & Wilkins. _Study Guide to Accompany Essentials of Nursing Research_, by Denise F. Polit and Cheryl Tatano Beck.

b. Is this a qualitative or quantitative study?

_____

_____

c. What is the underlying paradigm of the research?

_____

_____

d. Does the study involve the collection of empirical evidence?

_____

_____

e. Is the purpose of this study identification, description, exploration, explanation, and/or prediction and control?

_____

_____

f. Is this study applied or basic research?

_____

_____

QUESTIONS FOR DISCUSSION

a. How relevant is this study to the actual practice of nursing?

_____

_____

b. Could this study have been conducted as *either* a quantitative or qualitative study? Why or why not?

_____

_____

c. Which of the two studies cited in these exercises (the one in Appendix A or the one in Appendix B) is of greater interest and/or relevance to you personally? Why?

_____

_____

Copyright © 2006. Lippincott Williams & Wilkins. *Study Guide to Accompany Essentials of Nursing Research*, by Denise F. Polit and Cheryl Tatano Beck.

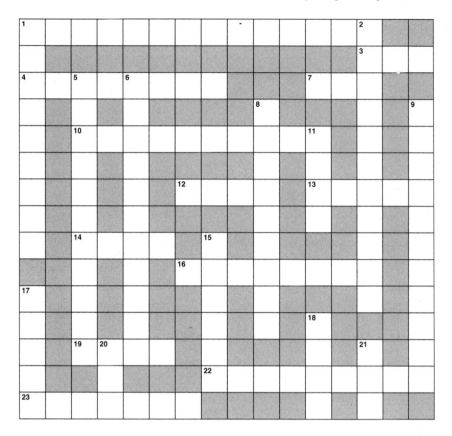

ACROSS

1. Nurses are increasingly encouraged to develop a practice that is _____ (hyphenated).

3. The clinical learning strategy developed at the McMaster School of Medicine (acronym)

4. A world view, a way of looking at natural phenomena

7. The world view that holds that there are multiple interpretations of reality (abbr.)

10. The world view that assumes that there is an orderly reality that can be studied objectively

12. The precursor to the National Institute of Nursing Research (acronym)

13. Successively trying alternative solutions is known as _____ and error.

14. Research designed to solve a pressing practical problem is _____ research (abbr.).

Copyright © 2006. Lippincott Williams & Wilkins. *Study Guide to Accompany Essentials of Nursing Research*, by Denise F. Polit and Cheryl Tatano Beck.

16. Research designed to document the effectiveness of health care services is _____ research.

19. The U.S. agency that promotes and sponsors nursing research (acronym)

22. A source of evidence reflecting ingrained customs

23. The _____ of nursing research began with Florence Nightingale.

DOWN

1. Evidence that is rooted in objective reality and gathered through the senses

2. The assumption that phenomena are not random, but rather have antecedent causes

5. The repeating of a study to determine if findings can be upheld with a new group of people

6. A purpose of doing research, involving a portrayal of phenomena as they exist

8. A scheme for ordering the utility of evidence for practice is an evidence _____.

9. A purpose of doing research, often linked to theory in quantitative studies

11. The techniques used by researchers to structure a study are called research _____ (abbr.).

15. The type of research that analyzes narrative, subjective materials is _____ research (abbr.).

17. An important nursing research journal, established in the 1970s (acronym)

18. The use of findings from research in a practice setting is called research _____ (abbr.).

20. A systematic review that amasses comprehensive research information is an _____ review (abbr.).

21. The U.S. agency within which NINR is housed (acronym)

Copyright © 2006. Lippincott Williams & Wilkins. *Study Guide to Accompany Essentials of Nursing Research,* by Denise F. Polit and Cheryl Tatano Beck.

CHAPTER 2

Comprehending Key Concepts in Qualitative and Quantitative Research

■ A. Matching Exercises

1. *Match each term in Set B with one of the responses in Set A. Indicate the letter corresponding to your response next to each item in Set B.*

SET A

a. Term used in quantitative research

b. Term used in qualitative research

c. Term used in both qualitative and quantitative research

SET B	RESPONSES
1. Subject	_____
2. Study participant	_____
3. Informant	_____
4. Variable	_____
5. Phenomena	_____
6. Construct	_____
7. Theory	_____
8. Data	_____
9. Bias	_____
10. Credibility	_____
11. Research control	_____
12. Generalizability	_____
13. Reflexivity	_____
14. Thick description	_____
15. Triangulation	_____

Copyright © 2006. Lippincott Williams & Wilkins. *Study Guide to Accompany Essentials of Nursing Research*, by Denise F. Polit and Cheryl Tatano Beck.

2. *Match each statement in Set B with one of the terms in Set A. Indicate the letter corresponding to your response next to each item in Set B.*

SET A

a. Independent variable

b. Dependent variable

c. Both independent and dependent variable

d. Neither independent nor dependent variable

SET B   **RESPONSES**

1. The variable that is the presumed effect   _____

2. The variable involved in a cause-and-effect relationship   _____

3. The variable that is the presumed cause   _____

4. The variable that is extraneous   _____

5. The variable, "length of stay in hospital"   _____

6. The variable that requires an operational definition   _____

7. The variable that is the main outcome of interest
   in the study   _____

8. The variable that is constant   _____

■ B. Completion Exercises

Write the words or phrases that correctly complete the sentences below.

1. In quantitative studies, the people who are being studied are often referred to as _____ ; they may be referred to as _____ _____ in both qualitative and quantitative studies.

2. The abstract qualities in which a researcher is interested are referred to by both qualitative and quantitative researchers as _____.

3. A _____, a term used primarily in quantitative research, is a quality of a person, group, setting, or situation that takes on different values.

4. The variable presumed to *cause* or influence changes in some other variable is the _____ variable.

Copyright © 2006. Lippincott Williams & Wilkins. *Study Guide to Accompany Essentials of Nursing Research*, by Denise F. Polit and Cheryl Tatano Beck.

5. The variable that the researcher wants to understand, explain, or predict is known as the _____ variable or the _____ variable.

6. If a researcher studied the effect of a scheduling assignment on nurses' morale, the scheduling assignment would be the _____ variable.

7. A variable that is irrelevant in a quantitative investigation and needs to be controlled is called a(n) _____ variable.

8. The pieces of information obtained in the course of a study are collectively known as the _____.

9. Quantitative researchers carefully specify how to measure concepts of interest, resulting in _____.

10. When the data are in the form of narrative descriptions, the data are _____ _____.

11. While quantitative researchers are often interested in studying relationships between variables, qualitative researchers examine _____.

12. "The higher the daily caloric intake, the greater the weight" expresses a presumed _____ relationship.

13. The process of developing generalizations from specific observations is referred to as _____ reasoning.

14. The process of developing specific predictions from general principles is _____ _____ reasoning.

15. Two important criteria for evaluating the quality of quantitative studies are _____ _____ and _____.

16. In qualitative research, the worth of the study can be evaluated through assessments of its _____.

17. When researchers use multiple referents to draw conclusions, they are using _____.

18. In thinking about how research findings can be used in other settings or contexts, quantitative researchers are concerned about _____ and qualitative researchers are concerned about _____.

Copyright © 2006. Lippincott Williams & Wilkins. *Study Guide to Accompany Essentials of Nursing Research*, by Denise F. Polit and Cheryl Tatano Beck.

■ C. Study Questions

1. Complete the crossword puzzle at the end of the chapter, which uses terms and concepts presented in Chapter 2. (Puzzles may be removed for easier viewing.)

2. Suggest operational definitions for the following concepts:

   a. Stress:

   _____

   _____

   b. Prematurity of infants:

   _____

   _____

   c. Fatigue:

   _____

   _____

   d. Pain:

   _____

   _____

   e. Obesity:

   _____

   _____

   f. Prolonged labor:

   _____

   _____

   g. Smoking behavior:

   _____

   _____

3. In each of the following research questions, identify the independent and dependent variables.

   a. Does assertiveness training improve the effectiveness of psychiatric nurses?

   Independent: _____

   Dependent: _____

Copyright © 2006. Lippincott Williams & Wilkins. *Study Guide to Accompany Essentials of Nursing Research*, by Denise F. Polit and Cheryl Tatano Beck.

b. Does the postural positioning of patients affect their respiratory function?

Independent: _____

Dependent: _____

c. Is the psychological well-being of patients affected by the amount of touch received from nursing staff?

Independent: _____

Dependent: _____

d. Is the incidence of decubitus ulcers reduced by more frequent turnings of patients?

Independent: _____

Dependent: _____

e. Are people who were abused as children more likely than others to abuse their own children?

Independent: _____

Dependent: _____

f. Is tolerance for pain related to a patient's age and gender?

Independent: _____

Dependent: _____

g. Is the number of prenatal visits of pregnant women associated with labor and delivery outcomes?

Independent: _____

Dependent: _____

h. Are levels of depression higher among children who experience the death of a sibling than among other children?

Independent: _____

Dependent: _____

i. Is compliance with a medical regimen higher among women than among men?

Independent: _____

Dependent: _____

j. Is anxiety in surgical patients affected by structured preoperative teaching?

Independent: _____

Dependent: _____

Copyright © 2006. Lippincott Williams & Wilkins. *Study Guide to Accompany Essentials of Nursing Research*, by Denise F. Polit and Cheryl Tatano Beck.

k. Does participating in a support group enhance coping among family caregivers of AIDS patients?

Independent: _____

Dependent: _____

l. Is hearing acuity of the elderly affected by the time of day?

Independent: _____

Dependent: _____

m. Is patient satisfaction with nursing care related to the congruity of nurses' and patients' cultural backgrounds?

Independent: _____

Dependent: _____

n. Is a midlife woman's educational attainment related to the frequency of obtaining a mammogram?

Independent: _____

Dependent: _____

o. Does home birth affect the parents' satisfaction with the childbirth experience?

Independent: _____

Dependent: _____

4. Below is a list of variables. For each, think of a research problem for which the variable would be the independent variable, and a second for which the variable would be the dependent variable. For example, take the variable "birth weight of infants." We might ask, "Does the age of the mother affect the birth weight of her infant (dependent variable)?" Alternatively, another research question might be, "Does the birth weight of infants (independent variable) affect their sensorimotor development at 6 months of age?" HINT: For the dependent variable problem, ask yourself, What factors might affect, influence, or cause this variable? For the independent variable problem, ask yourself, What factors does this variable influence, cause, or affect?

a. Body temperature

Independent: _____

Dependent: _____

b. Amount of sleep

Independent: _____

Dependent: _____

Copyright © 2006. Lippincott Williams & Wilkins. *Study Guide to Accompany Essentials of Nursing Research*, by Denise F. Polit and Cheryl Tatano Beck.

c. Frequency of practicing breast self-examination

Independent: _____

Dependent: _____

d. Level of hopefulness in cancer patients

Independent: _____

Dependent: _____

e. Stress among victims of domestic violence

Independent: _____

Dependent: _____

5. Look at the table of contents of a recent issue of *Nursing Research* (available at www.nursingcenter.com/library) or *Research in Nursing & Health* (available at www.interscience.wiley.com). Pick out a study title (not looking at the abstract) that implies that a relationship between variables was studied. Indicate what you think the independent and dependent variables might be, and what the title suggests about the nature of the relationship (i.e., causal or not).

■ D. Application Exercise

1. Read the abstract and introduction (the material before "methods") to the study in Appendix C ("Older Men's Health"). Then answer the following questions:

QUESTIONS OF FACT

a. Who was the researcher and what are her credentials and affiliation?

_____

_____

b. Who were the study participants?

_____

_____

c. What is the independent variable (or variables) in this study? Is this variable *inherently* an independent variable?

_____

_____

Copyright © 2006. Lippincott Williams & Wilkins. *Study Guide to Accompany Essentials of Nursing Research*, by Denise F. Polit and Cheryl Tatano Beck.

d. What is the dependent variable (or variables) in this study? Is this variable *inherently* a dependent variable?

_____

_____

e. Did the introduction actually use the terms "independent variable" or "dependent variable"?

_____

_____

f. Were the data in this study quantitative or qualitative?

_____

_____

g. Were any relationships under investigation? What type of relationship?

_____

_____

h. Two important variables were "held constant" in this study—what were they?

_____

_____

i. Does anything in the abstract or introduction suggest that "randomness" was used as a strategy in this study?

_____

_____

QUESTIONS FOR DISCUSSION

a. How relevant is this study to the actual practice of nursing?

_____

_____

b. Could this study have been conducted as *either* a quantitative or qualitative study? Why or why not?

_____

_____

c. Discuss the issue of generalizability within the context of this study, based on the introductory materials. To whom would it be *inappropriate* to generalize the

Copyright © 2006. Lippincott Williams & Wilkins. *Study Guide to Accompany Essentials of Nursing Research*, by Denise F. Polit and Cheryl Tatano Beck.

ts of the study? Are the results of this study, conducted in the United States, ely to be generalizable to other countries?

_____

_____

Read the abstract and introduction (the material before the section "research design") to the study in Appendix D ("Empowerment Process"). Then answer the following questions:

QUESTIONS OF FACT

a. Who was the researcher and what are her credentials and affiliation?

_____

_____

b. Did the researcher receive funding that supported this research?

_____

_____

c. Who were the study participants?

_____

_____

d. What were the key concepts in this study?

_____

_____

e. Were the data in this study quantitative or qualitative?

_____

_____

f. In what type of setting did the study take place?

_____

_____

g. Were any relationships under investigation?

_____

_____

Copyright © 2006. Lippincott Williams & Wilkins. *Study Guide to Accompany Essentials of Nursing Research*, by Denise F. Polit and Cheryl Tatano Beck.

h. Did the researcher "hold constant" any variables?

_____

_____

i. Does anything in the abstract or introduction suggest that "randomness" was used as a strategy in this study?

_____

_____

QUESTIONS FOR DISCUSSION

a. How relevant is this study to the actual practice of nursing?

_____

_____

b. Could this study have been conducted as *either* a quantitative or qualitative study? Why or why not?

_____

_____

c. Discuss the issue of transferability within the context of this study, based on the introductory materials. Are there communities to whom it would be *inappropriate* to transfer the findings? Are the results of this study, conducted in the United States, likely to be transferable to other countries?

_____

_____

d. Which of the two studies cited in these exercises (the one in Appendix C or the one in Appendix D) is of greater interest and/or relevance to you personally? Why?

_____

_____

Copyright © 2006. Lippincott Williams & Wilkins. *Study Guide to Accompany Essentials of Nursing Research*, by Denise F. Polit and Cheryl Tatano Beck.

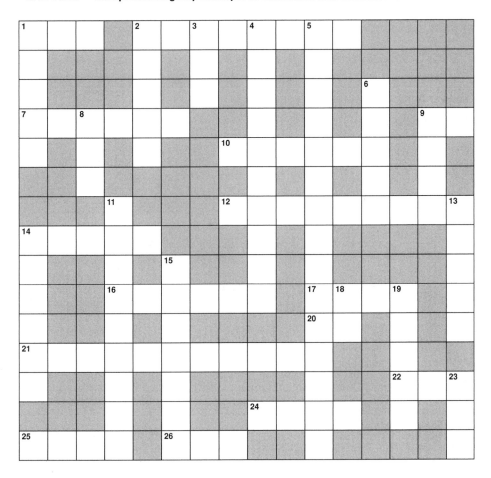

ACROSS

1. A relationship expresses a bond between at least _____ variables.

2. Study participants, in quantitative studies

7. In "What is the effect of diet on cancer?" the dependent variable is _____.

9. Example of a constant (mathematical construct)

10. A relationship in which one variable directly results in changes in another is a _____ relationship.

12. Another name for outcome variable is _____ variable.

14. In "What is the effect of radon on health?" the independent variable is _____.

16. An operational definition of nursing knowledge might be the _____ on the N-CLEX exam.

Copyright © 2006. Lippincott Williams & Wilkins. *Study Guide to Accompany Essentials of Nursing Research*, by Denise F. Polit and Cheryl Tatano Beck.

17. A distorting influence on study results

20. The cause of another variable (acronym)

21. The _____ definition indicates how a variable will be measured or observed.

22. The variables that are the effects (acronym)

24. Pieces of information gathered in a study

25. In 7 across, the independent variable

26. A formal, controlled setting for a study (abbr.)

DOWN

1. Qualitative researchers use _____ description to enhance the use of findings in other settings.

2. In "How does pain affect sleep?" the dependent variable is _____.

3. An operational definition of obesity (acronym—trick question!)

4. The variable that can confound understanding of relationships of interest

5. Analogous to generalizability, in qualitative studies

6. If quantitative study findings are convincing and well-grounded, they are likely to be _____.

8. Studies done in the field are done in _____ settings (abbr.).

9. In 2 down, the independent variable

11. A somewhat more complex abstraction than a concept

13. If a qualitative study is done with rigor, its findings are _____ worthy.

14. Quantitative researchers often design aspects of a study to happen by chance, or at _____.

15. Quantitative researchers often strive to exert research _____ over aspects of their studies.

18. The variable that influences another variable (acronym)

19. A research investigation

23. All the information in a study collectively comprises the data _____.

Copyright © 2006. Lippincott Williams & Wilkins. *Study Guide to Accompany Essentials of Nursing Research*, by Denise F. Polit and Cheryl Tatano Beck.

CHAPTER 3

Overview of the Research Process in Qualitative and Quantitative Studies

■ A. Matching Exercises

1. *Match each activity in Set B with one of the options in Set A. Indicate the letter corresponding to your response next to each item in Set B.*

SET A

a. An activity in quantitative research

b. An activity in qualitative research

c. An activity in both qualitative and quantitative research

d. An activity in neither quantitative nor qualitative research

SET B   **RESPONSES**

1. Choosing between an experimental or nonexperimental design   _____

2. Ending data collection once saturation has been achieved   _____

3. Developing or evaluating measuring instruments   _____

4. Doing a literature review   _____

5. Developing a sampling plan that ensures representativeness   _____

6. Taking steps to ensure protection of human rights   _____

7. Developing strategies to avoid data collection   _____

8. Disseminating research results   _____

9. Analyzing the data for major themes or categories   _____

10. Developing hypotheses to be tested statistically   _____

2. *Match each activity relating to quantitative studies in Set B with an option in Set A. Indicate the letter corresponding to your response next to each item in Set B.*

SET A

a. Conceptual phase

b. Planning phase

Copyright © 2006. Lippincott Williams & Wilkins. *Study Guide to Accompany Essentials of Nursing Research*, by Denise F. Polit and Cheryl Tatano Beck.

c. Empirical phase

d. Analytic phase

e. Dissemination phase

SET B	RESPONSES
1. Distributing questionnaires to a group of nursing home residents	_____
2. Deciding which extraneous variables need to be controlled	_____
3. Conducting a literature review	_____
4. Identifying a suitable theoretical framework	_____
5. Deciding to collect data from 300 alcoholics in treatment	_____
6. Determining what percentage of subjects were clinically depressed	_____
7. Presenting a paper at a meeting of the Eastern Nursing Research Society	_____
8. Designing a training session for data collectors	_____
9. Coding data for entry of information into a computer file	_____
10. Interpreting findings that were contrary to the hypotheses	_____

■ B. Completion Exercises

Write the words or phrases that correctly complete the sentences below.

1. In experimental research, researchers introduce a(n) _____, while this is not the case in nonexperimental research.

2. The three research traditions that have been especially fruitful among qualitative nurse researchers include _____, _____, and _____.

3. The research tradition that is concerned with *lived experience* and its meaning is

_____.

4. _____ seeks to describe and understand social psychological processes occurring in social settings.

5. There is typically a well-defined, prespecified set of activities with fairly linear progression in a _____ study.

6. Quantitative researchers may formulate predictions (_____) to be tested during the conceptual phase of the project.

Copyright © 2006. Lippincott Williams & Wilkins. *Study Guide to Accompany Essentials of Nursing Research,* by Denise F. Polit and Cheryl Tatano Beck.

7. If a research problem is clinical in nature, researchers can gain a better appreciation of clinical procedures, clients, and settings by engaging in _____ _____ before designing the study.

8. The overall plan for addressing a question through empirical investigation is called the _____.

9. The aggregate of people to whom researchers wish to generalize their results is the

    _____.

10. The actual group of people selected from a larger group to participate in a study is the

    _____.

11. The task of organizing and synthesizing the information collected in a study is known as _____.

12. A small-scale trial run of a research study is referred to as a(n) _____.

13. Study findings are communicated in a(n) _____.

14. The final phase of a research project is known as the _____ phase.

15. In a qualitative study, an important activity after identifying a research site is developing a strategy for _____ into selected settings within the site.

16. The individuals who control access to research sites or settings are known as the

    _____.

17. The design of a qualitative study is not predetermined before fieldwork begins; it is a(n) _____ design that responds to information as it is gathered.

18. Qualitative researchers' sampling decisions are often guided by the principle of

    _____ of the data.

■ C. Study Questions

1. Complete the crossword puzzle at the end of the chapter, which uses terms and concepts presented in Chapter 3. (Puzzles may be removed for easier viewing.)

2. Describe what is wrong with the following statements:

   a. Opitz's experimental study was conducted within the ethnographic tradition.

      _____

      _____

Copyright © 2006. Lippincott Williams & Wilkins. *Study Guide to Accompany Essentials of Nursing Research,* by Denise F. Polit and Cheryl Tatano Beck.

b. Brusser's experimental study examined the effect of relaxation therapy (the dependent variable) on pain (the independent variable) in cancer patients.

_____

_____

c. Ball's grounded theory study of the caregiving process for caretakers of patients with dementia controlled for the extraneous variables of patient age and gender.

_____

_____

d. In Meenan's phenomenological study of the meaning of futility among AIDS patients, subjects received an intervention designed to sustain hope.

_____

_____

e. In her experimental study, Gabris developed her data collection plan after she introduced her intervention to a group of patients.

_____

_____

3. Read the following report of a phenomenological study and identify segments of _raw data_: Evans, M. K. & O'Brien, B. (2005). Gestational diabetes: The meaning of an at-risk pregnancy. _Qualitative Health Research_, _15_, 66–81. Describe the effect that removal of the raw data would have on the report.

4. Which qualitative research tradition do you think would be most appropriate for the research questions below? Justify your response.

a. How do the health beliefs of Chinese immigrants influence their health-seeking behavior?

_____

_____

b. What is it like to be a recovering alcoholic?

_____

_____

c. What is the process by which widowers adapt to the sudden loss of their wives?

_____

_____

Copyright © 2006. Lippincott Williams & Wilkins. _Study Guide to Accompany Essentials of Nursing Research_, by Denise F. Polit and Cheryl Tatano Beck.

■ D. Application Exercises

1. Read the abstract and skim the report by Egan and coresearchers in Appendix E ("Nursing-Based Case Management"). Then answer the following questions:

QUESTIONS OF FACT

  a. What type of data was collected in this study—qualitative or quantitative?

  _____

  _____

  b. Could the study be described as an ethnographic, phenomenological, or grounded theory study?

  _____

  _____

  c. What is the paradigm underlying this study?

  _____

  _____

  d. Is this an experimental or nonexperimental study?

  _____

  _____

  e. What is the independent variable in this study?

  _____

  _____

  f. What were the dependent variables in this study?

  _____

  _____

  g. In the "method" section, what does the report say about the study design?

  _____

  _____

  h. Was the concept of "randomness" used in the design of this study?

  _____

  _____

Copyright © 2006. Lippincott Williams & Wilkins. *Study Guide to Accompany Essentials of Nursing Research*, by Denise F. Polit and Cheryl Tatano Beck.

i. Does the report describe an intervention? If so, what is it?

_____

_____

j. Did the report provide information about how key study variables were measured?

_____

_____

k. Did the study involve statistical analysis of data?

_____

_____

l. Did the study involve qualitative analysis of data?

_____

_____

m. Did the researchers disseminate their findings?

_____

_____

QUESTIONS FOR DISCUSSION

a. How relevant is this study to the actual practice of nursing?

_____

_____

b. Comment on why you think the research team collected both qualitative and quantitative data. What do you think would be the effect of omitting the quantitative data? Omitting the qualitative data?

_____

_____

c. The study was conducted in Australia. Comment on your view about how generalizable the results would be to other countries.

_____

_____

Copyright © 2006. Lippincott Williams & Wilkins. *Study Guide to Accompany Essentials of Nursing Research*, by Denise F. Polit and Cheryl Tatano Beck.

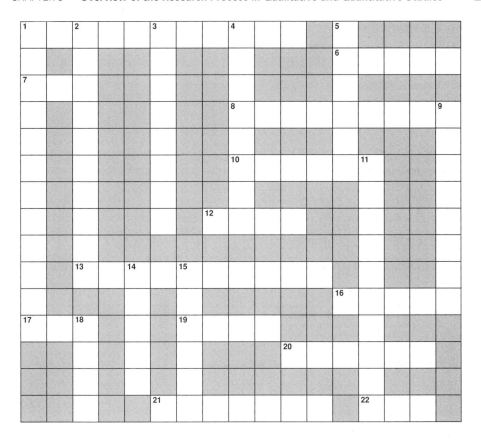

ACROSS

1. The qualitative tradition that focuses on the study of cultures

6. The type of design used in qualitative studies (abbr.)

7. The entire aggregate of units in which a researcher is interested (abbr.)

8. Qualitative studies are often undertaken within an underlying disciplinary _____.

10. The procedure of translating data into numerical values

12. A type of fieldwork done to enhance the value of a study for practicing nurses (abbr.)

13. A principle used to decide when to stop sampling in a qualitative study

16. When would an experiment involve an emergent design?

17. Quantitative researchers develop a knowledge context by doing a _____ review early in the project (abbr.).

19. Before selecting subjects, a quantitative researcher develops a sampling _____.

20. The subset of the population from whom information is gathered

Copyright © 2006. Lippincott Williams & Wilkins. *Study Guide to Accompany Essentials of Nursing Research*, by Denise F. Polit and Cheryl Tatano Beck.

21. When planning their studies, both qualitative and quantitative researchers need to address _____ issues to protect study participants.

22. Data that are in the exact same form as when they were collected are _____ data.

DOWN

1. The type of research that involves an intervention

2. Quantitative researchers formulate _____, which state expectations about how variables are related.

3. A qualitative tradition that focuses on social psychological processes within a social setting is _____ theory.

4. A step in experimental research is the development of an intervention _____.

5. The overall plan for obtaining answers to research questions is the research _____.

9. Quantitative research that observes and measures without intervening is called _____ (abbr.).

11. The individual with whom a researcher must negotiate to gain entrée into a site

14. Qualitative researchers begin with a broad _____ area to be studied.

15. In the dissemination phase, researchers prepare a research _____.

18. The empirical phase of a study typically requires a lot of _____.

Copyright © 2006. Lippincott Williams & Wilkins. *Study Guide to Accompany Essentials of Nursing Research*, by Denise F. Polit and Cheryl Tatano Beck.

CHAPTER 4

Reading Research Reports

■ A. Matching Exercises

1. *Match each statement from Set B with one of the sections in a research report, as listed in Set A. Indicate the letter corresponding to your response next to each item in Set B.*

SET A

a. Abstract

b. Introduction

c. Method

d. Results

e. Discussion

SET B   **RESPONSES**

1. Describes the research design   _____

2. In quantitative studies, presents outcomes of statistical analyses   _____

3. Identifies the research questions or hypotheses   _____

4. Presents a brief summary of the major features of the study   _____

5. Provides information on study participants and how they were selected   _____

6. Offers an interpretation of the study findings   _____

7. In qualitative studies, describes the themes that emerged from the data   _____

8. Offers a rationale for the study and describes its significance   _____

9. Describes how the research data were collected   _____

10. Identifies the study's main limitations   _____

11. This sentence would appear there: "The purpose of this study was to explore the process by which patients cope with a cancer diagnosis."   _____

12. In qualitative reports, includes raw data in the form of excerpts   _____

Copyright © 2006. Lippincott Williams & Wilkins. *Study Guide to Accompany Essentials of Nursing Research*, by Denise F. Polit and Cheryl Tatano Beck.

■ B. Completion Exercises

Write the words or phrases that correctly complete the sentences below.

1. Research findings summarized at a professional conference can be presented in one of two formats: _____ or _____.

2. The type of research reports that students are most likely to read are _____ _____.

3. The _____ of a research report succinctly conveys to prospective readers what was studied and what was learned.

4. Traditional abstracts are a single summary paragraph, but the "new style" abstracts are somewhat longer and have specific _____.

5. In a qualitative research report, the _____ would describe the central phenomenon under study.

6. "The data were collected by conducting face-to-face interviews with a sample of 100 nursing home residents" is a sentence most likely to appear in the _____ _____ section of a research report.

7. A(n) _____ is a procedure used in quantitative studies for testing hypotheses and evaluating the believability of the results.

8. In statistical testing, the _____ indicates how probable it is that the findings are reliable.

9. In a qualitative report, results are often organized according to major _____ _____.

10. The following sentence would most likely appear in the _____ section of a research report: "These findings suggest that women who are physically abused are more likely to suffer from depression and fatigue than nonabused women."

■ C. Study Questions

1. Complete the crossword puzzle at the end of the chapter, which uses terms and concepts presented in Chapter 4. (Puzzles may be removed for easier viewing.)

Copyright © 2006. Lippincott Williams & Wilkins. *Study Guide to Accompany Essentials of Nursing Research*, by Denise F. Polit and Cheryl Tatano Beck.

2. Why are qualitative research reports generally easier to read than quantitative research reports?

_____

_____

_____

_____

_____

3. Read the following abstract and rewrite it as a "new style" abstract with specific headings (Dixon, D., & Saul, J. [2003]. HIV sexual risk behavior among Puerto Rican women. *Health Care Women International, 24,* 529–543):

We examined the association of primary or nonprimary sexual partner relationship status on sexual risk behaviors, including condom use, among Latina women who are at self-disclosed increased heterosexual risk for human immunodeficiency virus (HIV) infection. Data were collected via structured interviews of 187 Puerto Rican women, aged 18–35, who attended a health clinic in the Bronx, New York. Approximately 13% of participants reported sexual activities with both primary and nonprimary sexual partners during the 6 months prior to the interview. Primary or nonprimary sexual partner status was associated with significant differences in frequency of condom use during anal sex and oral-penile sex, with more frequent condom use reported during these sexual activities with nonprimary sexual partners. Thus, potential contextual differences associated with primary or nonprimary relationship status may represent important factors to consider when designing interventions to facilitate HIV-protective behaviors among populations of urban women identified at increased heterosexual risk for HIV infection.

4. Read the titles of the journal articles appearing in the February 2005 issue of *Applied Nursing Research* (or some other issue of this journal). Evaluate the titles of the articles in terms of length and adequacy in communicating essential information about the studies.

5. Below is a brief abstract of a fictitious study, followed by a critique. Do you agree with the critique? Can you add other comments relevant to issues discussed in Chapter 4 of the textbook?

Fictitious Study. Guslander (2005) prepared the following abstract for her study:

Family members often experience considerable anxiety while their loved ones are in surgery. This study examined the effectiveness of a nursing intervention that involved providing oral intraoperative progress reports to family members. Surgical patients undergoing elective procedures were selected to either have family members receive the intervention or not have them receive it. The findings indicated that the family members in the intervention group were less anxious than family members who received the usual care.

Critique. This brief abstract provides a general overview of the nature of Guslander's study. It indicates a rationale for the study (the high anxiety level of surgical patients' family members) and summarizes what the researcher did. However, the abstract

Copyright © 2006. Lippincott Williams & Wilkins. *Study Guide to Accompany Essentials of Nursing Research,* by Denise F. Polit and Cheryl Tatano Beck.

could well have provided more information while still staying within a 200-word guideline (the abstract only contains 75 words). For example, the abstract could have better described the nature of the intervention (e.g., At what point during the operation was information given to family members? How much detail was provided? etc.). For a reader to have a preliminary assessment of the worth of the study—and therefore to make a decision about whether to read the entire report—more information about the methods would also have been helpful. For example, the abstract should have indicated such methodologic features as how the researcher measured anxiety and how many surgical patients were in the sample. Some indication of the study's implications would also have enhanced the usefulness of the abstract.

■ D. Application Exercises

1. Skim the study by Gibbins and coresearchers in Appendix A ("Procedural Pain"). Then answer the following questions:

QUESTIONS OF FACT

  a. Does the structure of this report follow the IMRAD format?

  _____

  _____

  b. Is the abstract a traditional narrative or is it a "new style" abstract?

  _____

  _____

  c. Does the abstract include information about the study purpose, how the study was done, what the findings were, and what the findings mean?

  _____

  _____

  d. Skim the method section. Is the presentation in the active or passive voice?

  _____

  _____

  e. Is this study experimental or nonexperimental?

  _____

  _____

Copyright © 2006. Lippincott Williams & Wilkins. *Study Guide to Accompany Essentials of Nursing Research,* by Denise F. Polit and Cheryl Tatano Beck.

QUESTIONS FOR DISCUSSION

a. What parts of the abstract were most difficult to understand? Identify words that you consider to be research "jargon."

_____

_____

b. Comment on the organization *within* the method section of this report.

_____

_____

2. Skim the study by Rew in Appendix B ("Homeless Youth"). Then answer the following questions:

QUESTIONS OF FACT

a. Does the structure of this report follow the IMRAD format?

_____

_____

b. Is the abstract a traditional narrative or is it a "new style" abstract?

_____

_____

c. Does the abstract include information about the study purpose, how the study was done, what the findings were, and what the findings mean?

_____

_____

d. Skim the method section. Is the presentation in the active or passive voice?

_____

_____

e. Is the study in one of the three main qualitative traditions described in Chapter 3? If so, which tradition?

_____

_____

QUESTIONS FOR DISCUSSION

a. What parts of the abstract were most difficult to understand?

_____

_____

Copyright © 2006. Lippincott Williams & Wilkins. *Study Guide to Accompany Essentials of Nursing Research*, by Denise F. Polit and Cheryl Tatano Beck.

b. Comment on the organization *within* the results section of this report.

_____

_____

c. Compare the level of difficulty of the abstracts for the two studies used in these exercises—i.e., the one in Appendix A and the one in Appendix B. Why do you think the level of difficulty differs?

_____

_____

ACROSS

1. The type of tests used by quantitative researchers to assess the reliability of their results
5. The section of the report that summarizes the analyses
7. The section of the report that presents interpretations
8. The first major section of a research report
11. Technical terminology that often makes research reports difficult to read
13. The section of the report that describes what the researcher did to answer the research question
14. "The lived experience of caring for a dying spouse" is an example of this part of a report
16. The type of reviewers who typically make recommendations about reports published in journals
17. Readers who check to ensure comprehension are _____ readers.
19. Statistical results that do not have a high probability of being reliable (abbr.)
20. The analyses of research data yield _____.
21. One conventional _____ of significance is .05.

DOWN

1. If the probability of a statistical test were .001, the results would be highly _____.
2. The type of format used to structure most research reports (acronym)
3. There are dozens of statistical _____ available for analyzing quantitative data.
4. The type of reviews in which reviewers and researchers do not know each other's identity
6. A summary of a study appearing at the beginning of a report
9. Journal editors rely on _____ by reviewers to make publication decisions.
10. One of two types of sessions at conferences at which researchers present their findings
11. Research reports are most likely to be accessed as _____ articles.
12. Nursing research began in the 19th century _____ (Latin acronym!).
15. The discussion section presents the researcher's ideas about what the findings _____.
18. A manuscript for a research report is typically between _____ and 25 pages double-spaced.

Copyright © 2006. Lippincott Williams & Wilkins. *Study Guide to Accompany Essentials of Nursing Research*, by Denise F. Polit and Cheryl Tatano Beck.

CHAPTER 5

Reviewing the Ethical Aspects of a Nursing Study

■ A. Matching Exercises

1. *Match each description in Set B with one of the procedures used to protect human subjects listed in Set A. Indicate the letter corresponding to the appropriate response next to each entry in Set B.*

SET A

a. Freedom from harm or exploitation

b. Informed consent

c. Anonymity

d. Confidentiality

SET B   **RESPONSES**

1. A questionnaire distributed by mail bears an identification number in one corner. Respondents are assured their responses will not be individually divulged.   _____

2. Hospitalized children included in a study, and their parents, are told the study's aims and procedures. Parents are asked to sign an authorization.   _____

3. Respondents in a study in which the same respondents will complete questionnaires at two points in time are asked to place their own four-digit identification number on the questionnaires and to memorize the number. Respondents are assured their answers will remain private.   _____

4. Study participants in an in-depth study of family members' coping with a natural disaster renegotiate the terms of their participation at successive interviews.   _____

5. Women who recently had a mastectomy are studied in terms of psychological consequences. In the interview, sensitive questions are carefully worded. After the interview, debriefing with the respondent determines the need for psychological support.   _____

Copyright © 2006. Lippincott Williams & Wilkins. *Study Guide to Accompany Essentials of Nursing Research*, by Denise F. Polit and Cheryl Tatano Beck.

6. Women interviewed in the above study (question 5) are told that the information they provide will not be individually divulged. _____

7. Subjects who volunteered for an experimental treatment for AIDS are warned of potential side effects and are asked to sign a waiver. _____

8. After determining that a new intervention resulted in subject discomfort, the researcher discontinues the study. _____

9. Unmarked questionnaires are distributed to a class of nursing students. The instructions indicate that responses will not be individually divulged. _____

10. The researcher assures subjects that they will be interviewed at a single point in time and adheres to this promise. _____

11. A questionnaire distributed to a sample of nursing students includes a statement indicating that completion and submission of the questionnaire will be construed as voluntary participation in a study. _____

12. The names, ages, and occupations of study participants whose interviews are excerpted in the research report are not divulged. _____

■ B. Completion Exercises

Write the words or phrases that correctly complete the sentences below.

1. Ethical _____ arise when participants' rights and the demands for rigorous evidence are put in direct conflict.

2. One of the first internationally recognized efforts to establish ethical standards was the

   _____.

3. In the United States, the National Commission for the Protection of Human Subjects of Biomedical and Behavioral Research issued a well-known set of guidelines known as the _____.

4. The most straightforward ethical precept is the protection of subjects from _____

   _____.

5. Risks that are no greater than those ordinarily encountered in daily life are referred to as _____.

6. The right to _____ means that prospective subjects have the right to voluntarily decide whether to participate in a study, without risk of penalty.

Copyright © 2006. Lippincott Williams & Wilkins. *Study Guide to Accompany Essentials of Nursing Research,* by Denise F. Polit and Cheryl Tatano Beck.

7. Researchers adhere to the principle of _____ by fully describing to participants the nature of the study and the likely risks and benefits of participation.

8. When researchers cannot link research information to the people who provided it, the condition known as _____ has prevailed.

9. Special procedures are often required to safeguard the rights of _____ _____ subjects.

10. Committees established in institutions to review proposed research procedures with respect to their adherence to ethical guidelines are often called IRBs, or _____ _____.

11. _____ cannot be achieved if participants are coerced or if they cannot understand the risks.

12. The three main issues covered in the official definition of *research misconduct* are _____, _____, and _____.

■ C. Study Questions

1. Complete the crossword puzzle at the end of the chapter, which uses terms and concepts presented in Chapter 5. (Puzzles may be removed for easier viewing.)

2. Below are descriptions of several research studies. Suggest some ethical dilemmas that are likely to emerge for each.

   a. A study of coping behaviors among rape victims

   _____

   _____

   b. An unobtrusive observational study of fathers' behaviors in the delivery room

   _____

   _____

   c. An interview study of the determinants of heroin addiction

   _____

   _____

   d. A study of dependence among mentally retarded children

   _____

   _____

Copyright © 2006. Lippincott Williams & Wilkins. *Study Guide to Accompany Essentials of Nursing Research,* by Denise F. Polit and Cheryl Tatano Beck.

e. An investigation of verbal interactions among schizophrenic patients

_____

_____

f. A study of the effects of a new drug on humans

_____

_____

3. The following two studies involved the use of vulnerable subjects. Evaluate the ethical aspects of one or both of these studies, paying special attention to the manner in which the subjects' heightened vulnerability was handled.

Shyu, Y. L. (2002). A conceptual framework for understanding the process of family caregiving to frail elders in Taiwan. *Research in Nursing & Health, 25*, 111–121.

Wise, B. V. (2002). In their own words: The lived experience of pediatric liver transplantation. *Qualitative Health Research, 12*, 74–90.

4. In the textbook, two actual studies with ethical problems were described (the study of syphilis among black men and the study in which live cancer cells were injected in elderly patients). Identify which ethical principles were transgressed in these studies.

_____

_____

_____

_____

_____

5. A stipend of $15 was paid to the women who completed a questionnaire concerning their sexual histories and other topics in the following study:

Kenney, J. W., Reinholtz, C., & Angelini, P. J. (1998). Sexual abuse, sex before age 16, and high-risk behaviors of your females with sexually transmitted disease. *Journal of Obstetric, Gynecologic, and Neonatal Nursing, 27*, 54–63.

Read the introductory sections of the report and comment on the appropriateness of the stipend.

6. Below is a brief description of the ethical aspects of a fictitious study, followed by a critique. Do you agree with the critique? Can you add other comments relevant to the ethical dimensions of the study?

Fictitious Study. Fortune conducted an in-depth study of nursing home patients to determine if their perceptions about personal control over decision making differed from the perceptions of the nursing staff. The investigator studied 25 nurse–patient dyads to determine whether there were differing perceptions and experiences regarding control over activities of daily living, such as arising, eating, and dressing. All of the nurses in the study were employed by the nursing home in which the patients resided. Because the

Copyright © 2006. Lippincott Williams & Wilkins. *Study Guide to Accompany Essentials of Nursing Research,* by Denise F. Polit and Cheryl Tatano Beck.

nursing home had no IRB, Fortune sought permission to conduct the study from the nursing home administrator. She also obtained the consent of the legal guardian or responsible family member of each patient. All study participants were fully informed about the nature of the study. The researcher assured the nurses and the legal guardians and family members of the patients of the confidentiality of the information and obtained their consent in writing. Data were gathered primarily through in-depth interviews with the patients and the nurses, at separate times. The researcher also observed interactions between the patients and nurses. The findings from the study showed that patients perceived that they had more control over all aspects of the activities of daily living (except eating) than the nurses perceived that they had. Excerpts from the interviews were used verbatim in the research report, but Fortune did not divulge the location of the nursing home, and she used fictitious names for all participants.

Critique. Fortune did a reasonably good job of adhering to basic ethical principles in the conduct of her research. She obtained written permission to conduct the study from the nursing home administrator, and she obtained informed consent from the nurse participants and the legal guardians or family members of the patients. The study participants were not put at risk in any way, and the patients who participated may actually have enjoyed the opportunity to have a conversation with the researcher. Fortune also took appropriate steps to maintain the confidentiality of participants. It is still unclear, however, whether the patients knowingly and willingly participated in the research. Nursing home residents are a vulnerable group. They may not have been aware of their right to refuse to be interviewed without fear of repercussion. Fortune could have enhanced the ethical aspects of the study by taking more vigorous steps to obtain the informed, voluntary consent of the nursing home residents or to exclude patients who could not reasonably be expected to understand the researcher's request. Given the vulnerability of the group, Fortune might also have established her own review panel composed of peers and interested lay people to review the ethical dimensions of her project. Debriefing sessions with study participants also would have been appropriate.

■ D. Application Exercises

1. Read the "procedures" subsection in the method section of the report by Gibbins and her colleagues ("Procedural Pain") in Appendix A. Then answer the following questions:

QUESTIONS OF FACT

a. Does the report indicate that the study procedures were reviewed by an IRB or other similar institutional human subjects group?

_____

_____

Copyright © 2006. Lippincott Williams & Wilkins. *Study Guide to Accompany Essentials of Nursing Research*, by Denise F. Polit and Cheryl Tatano Beck.

b. Would the subjects in this study be considered "vulnerable subjects"?

_____

_____

c. Were participants subjected to any physical harm or discomfort or psychological distress *as part of the study*? What efforts did the researchers make to minimize harm and maximize good?

_____

_____

d. Were participants (or their parents) deceived in any way?

_____

_____

e. Were participants coerced into participating in the study?

_____

_____

f. Were appropriate informed consent procedures used? Was there full disclosure, and was participation voluntary?

_____

_____

g. Does the report discuss steps that were taken to protect the privacy and confidentiality of study participants?

_____

_____

QUESTIONS FOR DISCUSSION

a. Do you think the benefits of this research outweighed the costs to participants— what is the overall risk/benefit ratio? Would you characterize the study as having *minimal risk*?

_____

_____

b. Do you think that the researchers took adequate steps to protect the study participants? If not, what else could they have done?

_____

_____

Copyright © 2006. Lippincott Williams & Wilkins. *Study Guide to Accompany Essentials of Nursing Research*, by Denise F. Polit and Cheryl Tatano Beck.

c. The report does not indicate that the subjects or their parents were paid a stipend. Should they have been, in your opinion?

_____

_____

2. Read the "procedure" subsection in the method section of the report by Rew ("Homeless Youth") in Appendix B. Then answer the following questions:

QUESTIONS OF FACT

a. Does the report indicate that the study procedures were reviewed by an IRB or other similar institutional human subjects group?

_____

_____

b. Would the study participants in this study be considered "vulnerable subjects"?

_____

_____

c. Were participants subjected to any physical harm or discomfort or psychological distress as part of this study? What efforts did the researchers make to minimize harm and maximize good?

_____

_____

d. Were participants deceived in any way?

_____

_____

e. Were participants coerced into participating in the study?

_____

_____

f. Were appropriate informed consent procedures used? Was there full disclosure, and was participation voluntary?

_____

_____

Copyright © 2006. Lippincott Williams & Wilkins. *Study Guide to Accompany Essentials of Nursing Research*, by Denise F. Polit and Cheryl Tatano Beck.

g. Does the report discuss steps that were taken to protect the privacy and confidentiality of study participants?

_____

_____

QUESTIONS FOR DISCUSSION

a. Do you think the benefits of this research outweighed the costs to participants—what is the overall risk/benefit ratio? Would you characterize the study as having *minimal risk*?

_____

_____

b. Do you think that the researchers took adequate steps to protect the study participants? If not, what else could they have done?

_____

_____

c. The report indicates that the study participants were paid a stipend. Comment on whether you think the stipend and the amount were appropriate.

_____

_____

Copyright © 2006. Lippincott Williams & Wilkins. *Study Guide to Accompany Essentials of Nursing Research*, by Denise F. Polit and Cheryl Tatano Beck.

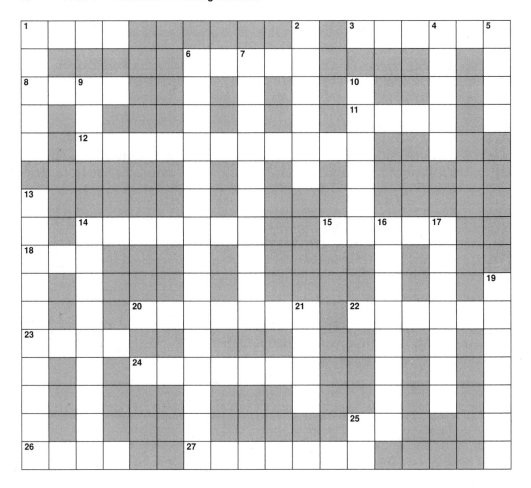

ACROSS

1. A fundamental right for study participants is freedom from _____.

3. Involves changing or omitting data or distorting results (abbr.)

6. Most disciplines have developed _____ of ethics.

8. Anonymity is a method of protecting this (abbr.).

11. Researchers should conduct a _____-benefit assessment.

12. A major ethical principle concerning maximizing benefits of research

14. The type of consent procedure that may be required in qualitative research

15. A young _____ is usually considered a vulnerable subject.

18. Debriefings give participants an opportunity to _____ complaints.

Copyright © 2006. Lippincott Williams & Wilkins. *Study Guide to Accompany Essentials of Nursing Research*, by Denise F. Polit and Cheryl Tatano Beck.

20. A payment sometimes offered to participants as an incentive to take part in a study

22. Data collection without participants' awareness, using concealment

23. A procedure for collecting data without linking them to individual participants (abbr.)

24. The report that is the basis for ethical regulations for studies funded by the U.S. government

25. Numbers used in place of names to protect individual identities (abbr.)

26. Fraud and misrepresentations are examples of research _____ (abbr.).

27. A major ethical principle involves respect for human _____ (reversed!).

DOWN

1. Legislation passed in the United States in 1996 concerning privacy (acronym)

2. Informal agreement to participate in a study (e.g., by minors)

4. The Declaration of Hel _____, the code of ethics of the World Medical Association

5. The ethical principle of *justice* includes the right to _____ treatment.

6. Participants' privacy is often protected by these procedures, even though the researchers know participants' identities.

7. People can make informed decisions about research participation when there is full _____.

9. A committee (in the United States) that reviews the ethical aspects of a study (acronym)

10. A situation in which private information is accidentally divulged is a _____ of confidentiality.

13. The appropriation of someone's words or ideas without proper credit

14. A vulnerable, institutionalized group with diminished autonomy

16. Most studies adhere to the practice of obtaining written _____ consent.

17. A conflict between the rights of participants and the demands for rigorous research creates an ethical _____.

19. Research that adheres to _____ guidelines is designed to protect participants' rights.

21. Mismanagement of _____ can result in a type of research misconduct.

Copyright © 2006. Lippincott Williams & Wilkins. *Study Guide to Accompany Essentials of Nursing Research*, by Denise F. Polit and Cheryl Tatano Beck.

PART 2

Preliminary Steps in the Research Process

CHAPTER 6

Scrutinizing Research Problems, Research Questions, and Hypotheses

■ A. Matching Exercises

1. *Match each description in Set B with one of the phrases listed in Set A. Indicate the letter corresponding to your response next to each entry in Set B.*

SET A

a. Statement of purpose—qualitative study

b. Statement of purpose—quantitative study

c. Not a statement of purpose for a research study

SET B   RESPONSES

1. The purpose of this study is to test whether the removal of physical restraints affects behavioral changes in elderly patients.   _____

2. The purpose of this project is to facilitate the transition from hospital to home among women who have just given birth.   _____

3. The goal of this project is to explore the process by which an elderly person adjusts to placement in a nursing home.   _____

4. The investigation was designed to document the incidence and prevalence of smoking, alcohol use, and drug use among adolescents aged 12 to 14.   _____

5. The study's purpose was to describe the nature of touch used by parents with their preterm infants.   _____

6. The goal is to develop guidelines for spiritually related nursing interventions.   _____

7. The purpose of this project is to examine the relationship between race/ethnicity and the use of over-the-counter medications.   _____

8. The purpose is to develop an in-depth understanding of patients' feelings of powerlessness in hospital settings.   _____

Copyright © 2006. Lippincott Williams & Wilkins. *Study Guide to Accompany Essentials of Nursing Research*, by Denise F. Polit and Cheryl Tatano Beck.

2. *Match each description in Set B with one of the phrases listed in Set A. Indicate the letter corresponding to your response next to each entry in Set B.*

SET A

a. Research hypothesis—directional

b. Research hypothesis—nondirectional

c. Null hypothesis

d. Not a hypothesis as stated

SET B   RESPONSES

1. First-born infants have higher concentrations of estrogens and progesterone in umbilical cord blood than do later-born infants. _____

2. There is no relationship between participation in prenatal classes and the health outcomes of infants. _____

3. Nursing students are increasingly interested in obtaining advanced degrees. _____

4. Nurse practitioners have more job mobility than do other registered nurses. _____

5. A person's age is related to his or her difficulty in accessing health care. _____

6. Glaucoma can be effectively screened by means of tonometry. _____

7. Higher noise levels result in increased anxiety among hospitalized patients. _____

8. Media exposure regarding the health hazards of smoking is unrelated to the public's smoking habits. _____

9. Patients' compliance with their medication regimens is related to their perceptions of the consequences of noncompliance. _____

10. The primary reason that nurses participate in continuing education programs is for professional advancement. _____

11. Nursing graduates from the United States and Canada differ with respect to their level of job satisfaction in their first nursing jobs. _____

12. A cancer patient's degree of hopefulness regarding the future is unrelated to his or her religiosity. _____

13. The degree of attachment between infants and their mothers is associated with the infant's status as low birth weight or normal birth weight. _____

Copyright © 2006. Lippincott Williams & Wilkins. *Study Guide to Accompany Essentials of Nursing Research*, by Denise F. Polit and Cheryl Tatano Beck.

14. The presence of homonymous hemianopia in stroke patients negatively affects their length of stay in hospital.   _____

15. Adjustment to hemodialysis does not vary by the patient's gender.   _____

■ B. Completion Exercises

Write the words or phrases that correctly complete the sentences below.

1. A(n) _____ is a situation involving an enigmatic, puzzling, or disturbing condition that is of interest to a researcher.

2. A(n) _____ is a statement of the specific query the researcher seeks to answer.

3. The accomplishments a researcher hopes to achieve by conducting a study are referred to as the _____ or _____.

4. The five most common sources of ideas for research problems are

   _____, _____, _____,

   _____, and _____.

5. Research questions involving the essence, experience, process, or nature of some phenomenon would likely be addressed in a _____ study.

6. Although it is desirable to have a statement of purpose placed early in a research report, the most typical location is at the end of the _____.

7. The part of speech that often communicates how researchers sought to address a research problem in a statement of purpose is _____.

8. Research hypotheses state a predicted _____ between variables.

9. A hypothesis involves a prediction regarding at least _____ variables.

10. Hypotheses predict the effect of the _____ variable on the _____ variable.

11. A hypothesis that states a prediction regarding two or more independent and two or more dependent variables is called a(n) _____ hypothesis.

12. The _____ hypothesis states that there is no expected relationship among the research variables.

Copyright © 2006. Lippincott Williams & Wilkins. *Study Guide to Accompany Essentials of Nursing Research*, by Denise F. Polit and Cheryl Tatano Beck.

■ C. Study Questions

1. Complete the crossword puzzle at the end of the chapter, which uses terms and concepts presented in Chapter 6. (Puzzles may be removed for easier viewing.)

2. Below is a list of general topics that could be investigated. Develop at least one research question for each, making sure that some are questions that could be addressed through qualitative research and others are ones that could be addressed through quantitative research. (HINT: For quantitative research questions, think of these concepts as potential independent or dependent variables, then ask, "What might cause or affect this variable?" and "What might be the consequences or effects of this variable?" This should lead to some ideas for research questions.)

   a. Patient comfort _____

   _____.

   b. Psychiatric patients' readmission rates _____

   _____.

   c. Anxiety in hospitalized children _____

   _____.

   d. Elevated blood pressure _____

   _____.

   e. Incidence of sexually transmitted diseases (STDs) _____

   _____.

   f. Patient cooperativeness in the recovery room _____

   _____.

   g. Caregiver stress _____

   _____.

   h. Mother–infant bonding _____

   _____.

   i. Menstrual irregularities _____

   _____.

Copyright © 2006. Lippincott Williams & Wilkins. *Study Guide to Accompany Essentials of Nursing Research*, by Denise F. Polit and Cheryl Tatano Beck.

3. Below are five nondirectional hypotheses. Restate each one as a directional hypothesis.

Nondirectional Hypothesis   *Directional Hypothesis*

a. Tactile stimulation is associated with
   comparable physiologic arousal as
   verbal stimulation among infants with
   congenital heart disease.

b. Nurses and patients differ in terms of
   the relative importance they attach to
   having the patients' physical versus
   emotional needs met.

c. Type of nursing care (primary versus
   team) is unrelated to patient
   satisfaction with the care received.

d. The incidence of decubitus ulcers is
   related to the age of the patient.

e. Nurses administer the same amount
   of narcotic analgesics to male and
   female patients.

4. Below are five simple hypotheses. Change each one to a complex hypothesis by
   adding either a dependent or independent variable.

Simple Hypothesis   *Complex Hypothesis*

a. First-time blood donors experience
   greater stress during the donation than
   donors who have given blood previously.

b. Nurses who initiate more conversation
   with patients are rated by patients as
   more effective in their nursing care than
   those who initiate less conversation.

Copyright © 2006. Lippincott Williams & Wilkins. *Study Guide to Accompany Essentials of Nursing Research*, by Denise F. Polit and Cheryl Tatano Beck.

c. Surgical patients who give high ratings
to the informativeness of nursing
communications experience less
preoperative anxiety than do patients
who give low ratings.

d. Appendectomy patients whose
peritoneums are drained with a
Jackson-Pratt drain will experience
more peritoneal infection than patients
who are not drained.

e. Women who give birth by cesarean
delivery are more likely to experience
postpartum depression than women
who give birth vaginally.

5. In study questions 3 and 4 above, 10 research hypotheses were provided. Identify the
independent and dependent variables in each.

INDEPENDENT VARIABLE(S)   **DEPENDENT VARIABLE(S)**

3a. _____   _____

3b. _____   _____

3c. _____   _____

3d. _____   _____

3e. _____   _____

4a. _____   _____

4b. _____   _____

4c. _____   _____

4d. _____   _____

4e. _____   _____

Copyright © 2006. Lippincott Williams & Wilkins. *Study Guide to Accompany Essentials of Nursing Research*, by Denise F. Polit and Cheryl Tatano Beck.

6. Below are five statements that are *not* research hypotheses as currently stated. Suggest modifications to these statements that would make them testable research hypotheses.

Original Statement   *Hypothesis*

a. Relaxation therapy is effective in reducing   _____

    hypertension.   _____

b. The use of bilingual health care staff   _____

    produces high utilization rates of health   _____

    care facilities by ethnic minorities.   _____

c. Nursing students are affected in their   _____

    choice of clinical specialization by   _____

    interactions with nursing faculty.   _____

d. Sexually active teenagers have a high   _____

    rate of using male methods of   _____

    contraception.   _____

e. In-use intravenous solutions become   _____

    contaminated within 48 hours.   _____

■ D. Application Exercises

1. Read the introduction to the report by Egan and colleagues ("Nursing-Based Case Management") in Appendix E. Then answer the following questions:

QUESTIONS OF FACT

a. In which paragraph of this report is the research problem stated? Summarize in two to three sentences what the problem is.

    _____

    _____

b. Does this report present a statement of purpose? If so, what *verb* do the researchers use in the statement, and is that verb consistent with the type of research that was undertaken?

    _____

    _____

Copyright © 2006. Lippincott Williams & Wilkins. *Study Guide to Accompany Essentials of Nursing Research*, by Denise F. Polit and Cheryl Tatano Beck.

c. Does the report specify a research question? If so, was it well-stated? If not, indicate what the research question was, as implied in the report.

_____

_____

d. Does the report specify hypotheses? If there are hypotheses, were they appropriately worded? Are they directional or nondirectional? Simple or complex? Research or null?

_____

_____

e. If no hypotheses were stated, what would one be?

_____

_____

f. Were hypotheses tested?

_____

_____

QUESTIONS FOR DISCUSSION

a. Did the researchers do an adequate job of describing the research problem?

_____

_____

b. Comment on the significance of the study's research problem for nursing.

_____

_____

c. Did the researchers do an adequate job of explaining the study's purpose, research questions, and/or hypotheses?

_____

_____

Copyright © 2006. Lippincott Williams & Wilkins. *Study Guide to Accompany Essentials of Nursing Research*, by Denise F. Polit and Cheryl Tatano Beck.

2. Read the introduction and "background" section of the report by Bent ("Empowerment Process") in Appendix D. Then answer the following questions:

QUESTIONS OF FACT

a. In which paragraph of this report is the research problem stated? Summarize in two to three sentences what the problem is.

_____

_____

b. Does this report present a statement of purpose? If so, what *verb* do the researchers use in the statement, and is that verb consistent with the type of research that was undertaken?

_____

_____

c. Does the report specify a research question? If so, was it well-stated? If not, indicate what the research question was, as implied in the report.

_____

_____

d. Does the report specify hypotheses? If there are hypotheses, were they appropriately worded? Are they directional or nondirectional? Simple or complex? Research or null?

_____

_____

e. If no hypotheses were stated, what would one be?

_____

_____

f. Were hypotheses tested?

_____

_____

QUESTIONS FOR DISCUSSION

a. Did the researchers do an adequate job of describing the research problem?

_____

_____

Copyright © 2006. Lippincott Williams & Wilkins. *Study Guide to Accompany Essentials of Nursing Research*, by Denise F. Polit and Cheryl Tatano Beck.

b. Comment on the significance of the study's research problem for nursing.

_____

_____

c. Did the researchers do an adequate job of explaining the study's purpose, research questions, and/or hypotheses?

_____

_____

Copyright © 2006. Lippincott Williams & Wilkins. *Study Guide to Accompany Essentials of Nursing Research*, by Denise F. Polit and Cheryl Tatano Beck.

ACROSS

5. A hypothesis in which the specific nature of the predicted relationship is not stipulated

7. Researchers express the disturbing situation in need of study in their problem _____.

8. A hypothesis stipulates the expected relationship between a(n) ___ and a DV (abbr.).

9. One phrase that indicates the relational aspect of a hypothesis is ___ than.

11. A topic for a research problem might arise from global _____ or political issues.

13. The name of a popular television series based on a hospital drama

15. One source of research problems, especially for hypothesis-testing research

16. A hypothesis with two or more independent and/or dependent variables

18. The results of hypothesis testing never constitute _____ that the hypotheses are or are not correct.

20. The purpose of a study is often conveyed through the judicious choice of _____.

21. A hypothesis must always involve at least _____ variables.

22. A statement of purpose indicating that the intent of the study was to *prove* or *demonstrate* something suggests a _____.

23. An interrogative wording of the study purpose

DOWN

1. A hypothesis with one independent and one dependent variable

2. The *actual* hypothesis of an investigator is the ___ hypothesis (abbr.).

3. Another name for *null* hypothesis

4. In complex hypotheses there are _____ independent or dependent variables

5. The hypothesis that posits no relationship between variables

6. A desired accomplishment in conducting a study

10. The researcher's overall goals of undertaking a study

12. A statement of the researcher's prediction about variables in the study (abbr.)

14. Hypotheses must predict a _____ between the independent and dependent variables (abbr.)

15. Hypotheses are typically put to a statistical _____.

17. A statement of _____ is a declaration that captures the general direction of the inquiry.

19. A research _____ is an enigmatic or troubling condition (abbr.).

Copyright © 2006. Lippincott Williams & Wilkins. *Study Guide to Accompany Essentials of Nursing Research*, by Denise F. Polit and Cheryl Tatano Beck.

CHAPTER 7

Finding and Reviewing Studies in the Literature

■ A. Matching Exercises

1. Match each statement in Set B with one of the types of literature review listed in Set A. Indicate the letter corresponding to your response next to each entry in Set B.

SET A

a. Traditional narrative review

b. Meta-analysis

c. Metasynthesis

d. All of the above

e. None of the above

SET B   **RESPONSES**

1. Most likely to be undertaken by students   _____

2. Uses statistical procedures   _____

3. Requires identifying and retrieving primary source material   _____

4. Integrates information from anecdotal reports   _____

5. A method of integrating qualitative studies   _____

6. Brief versions are in the introduction of most research reports   _____

7. Prepared by many practicing nurses   _____

8. Can be published as a stand-alone article in a research journal   _____

9. Relies primarily on searches through Internet search engines   _____

10. Is a totally objective approach to integrating study findings   _____

Copyright © 2006. Lippincott Williams & Wilkins. *Study Guide to Accompany Essentials of Nursing Research*, by Denise F. Polit and Cheryl Tatano Beck.

■ B. Completion Exercises

Write the words or phrases that correctly complete the sentences below.

1. For students who are just beginning to engage in their own research, the most important function of the literature review is likely to be as a source of _____.

2. The most important type of information to include in a research literature review is _____.

3. In the context of the research literature, a(n) _____ source is a description of a study written by the researchers who conducted it.

4. For nurses, the most widely used electronic database is _____.

5. Most electronic searches are likely to begin with a(n) _____ search.

6. An electronic search that looks for a topic or key word as it appears in the text fields of a record is referred to as a(n) _____ search.

7. The written literature review should paraphrase materials and use a minimum of _____.

8. The literature review should make clear not only what is known about a problem but also any _____ in the research.

9. The review should conclude with a(n) _____ of the available evidence.

10. The review should be written in a language of _____, in keeping with the limitations of available methods.

■ C. Study Questions

1. Complete the crossword puzzle at the end of the chapter, which uses terms and concepts presented in Chapter 7. (Puzzles may be removed for easier viewing.)

2. Below are several research questions. Indicate one or more key words that you would use to begin a literature search on this topic.

Research Questions   *Key Words*

   a. What is the lived experience of being a   _____

   survivor of a suicide attempt?   _____

Copyright © 2006. Lippincott Williams & Wilkins. *Study Guide to Accompany Essentials of Nursing Research*, by Denise F. Polit and Cheryl Tatano Beck.

   b. Does contingency contracting improve patient   _____

      compliance with a treatment regimen?   _____

   c. What is the decision-making process for a   _____

      woman considering having an abortion?   _____

   d. What is the process by which people make   _____

      decisions about going on a diet?   _____

   e. Is rehabilitation after spinal cord injury affected   _____

      by the patient's age and occupation?   _____

   f. What is the course of appetite loss among   _____

      cancer patients undergoing chemotherapy?   _____

   g. What is the effect of alcohol skin preparation   _____

      before insulin injection on the incidence   _____

      of local and systemic infection?   _____

   h. Are bottle-fed babies introduced to solid foods   _____

      sooner than breastfed babies?   _____

   i. Do children raised on vegetarian diets have   _____

      different growth patterns from other children?   _____

3. Below are fictitious excerpts from research literature reviews. Each excerpt has a stylistic problem. Change each sentence to make it acceptable stylistically.

Original   *Revised*

   a. Most elderly people do not eat a balanced   _____

      diet.   _____

   b. Patient characteristics have a significant impact   _____

      on nursing workload.   _____

   c. A child's conception of appropriate sick role   _____

      behavior changes as the child grows older.   _____

   d. Home birth poses many potential dangers.   _____

   e. Multiple sclerosis results in considerable   _____

      anxiety to the family of the patient.   _____

Copyright © 2006. Lippincott Williams & Wilkins. *Study Guide to Accompany Essentials of Nursing Research*, by Denise F. Polit and Cheryl Tatano Beck.

f. Studies have proved that most nurses prefer not to work the night shift.
_____
_____

g. Life changes are the major cause of stress in adults.
_____
_____

h. Stroke rehabilitation programs are most effective when they involve the patients' families.
_____
_____
_____

i. It has been proved that psychiatric outpatients have higher-than-average rates of accidental deaths and suicides.
_____
_____
_____

j. The traditional pelvic examination is sufficiently unpleasant to many women that they avoid having the examination.
_____
_____
_____

k. It is known that most tonsillectomies performed 3 decades ago were unnecessary.
_____
_____

l. Few smokers seriously try to break the smoking habit.
_____
_____

m. Severe cutaneous burns often result in hemorrhagic gastric erosions.
_____
_____

4. Read the Davidson et al. (2004) study entitled "Stressors and Self-Care Challenges Faced by Adolescents with Type 1 Diabetes," which appeared in *Applied Nursing Research, 17*, 72–80. Write a summary of the research problem, methods, findings, and conclusions of the study. Your summary should be capable of serving as notes for a review of the literature on stress among adolescents with diabetes.

5. Read the following research report (or another article of your choosing): Plach, S. K., Stevens, P. E., & Moss, V. A. (2004). Corporeality: Women's experience of a body with rheumatoid arthritis. *Clinical Nursing Research, 13*, 137–155. Complete as much information as you can about this report using the protocol in Figure 7-3.

6. Read the literature review section from a research article appearing in a nursing journal in the early 1990s (some possibilities are suggested below). Search the literature for more recent research on the topic of the article and update the original researchers' review section. Don't forget to incorporate in your review the findings from the cited research article itself! Here are some possible articles:

Copyright © 2006. Lippincott Williams & Wilkins. *Study Guide to Accompany Essentials of Nursing Research,* by Denise F. Polit and Cheryl Tatano Beck.

Bonheur, B., & Young, S. W. (1991). Exercise as a health-promoting lifestyle choice. *Applied Nursing Research, 4*, 2–6.

Long, K. A., & Boik, R. J. (1993). Predicting alcohol use in rural children. *Nursing Research, 42*, 79–86.

Morse, J. M., & Hutchinson, E. (1991). Releasing restraints: Providing safe care for the elderly. *Research in Nursing & Health, 14*, 382–396.

Quinn, M. M. (1991). Attachment between mothers and their Down syndrome infants. *Western Journal of Nursing Research, 13*, 382–396.

Singer, N. (1995). Understanding sexual risk behavior from drug users' accounts of their life experiences. *Qualitative Health Research, 5*, 237–249.

■ D. Application Exercises

1. Read the abstract, introduction, and first subsection under the method section of the report by Taylor-Piliae and Froelicher ("Effectiveness of Tai Chi") in Appendix F. Then answer the following questions:

QUESTIONS OF FACT

   a. What type of research review did the investigators undertake?

   _____

   _____

   b. Did the researchers begin with a problem statement? Summarize the problem in two to three sentences.

   _____

   _____

   c. Did the researchers provide a statement of purpose? If so, what was it?

   _____

   _____

   d. How many different databases did the researchers search? Were the searches of electronic databases? Were any manual methods used in the search?

   _____

   _____

   e. What key words were used in the search? Were the key words related to the independent or dependent variable of interest?

   _____

   _____

Copyright © 2006. Lippincott Williams & Wilkins. *Study Guide to Accompany Essentials of Nursing Research*, by Denise F. Polit and Cheryl Tatano Beck.

f. Did the researchers restrict their search to English-language reports?

_____

_____

g. How many citations were initially identified by the search?

_____

_____

h. Was there any redundancy in the citations retrieved from the various databases?

_____

_____

i. What are some of the reasons the researchers cited for eliminating some of the retrieved studies from further consideration?

_____

_____

j. How many studies ultimately were included in the review?

_____

_____

k. Were the studies included in the review qualitative, quantitative, or both?

_____

_____

QUESTIONS FOR DISCUSSION

a. Did the researchers do an adequate job of explaining the problem and the study purpose?

_____

_____

b. Did the researchers appear to do a thorough job in their search for relevant studies?

_____

_____

c. Certain studies that were initially retrieved were eliminated. Did the researchers provide a sound rationale for their decisions?

_____

_____

Copyright © 2006. Lippincott Williams & Wilkins. *Study Guide to Accompany Essentials of Nursing Research*, by Denise F. Polit and Cheryl Tatano Beck.

2. Read the following sections of the report by Beck ("Mothering Multiples") in Appendix G: the abstract, the section "What is Meta-Synthesis?" and the first paragraph under "A Meta-Synthesis of Qualitative Research on Mothering Multiples." Then answer the following questions:

QUESTIONS OF FACT

a. What type of research review did Beck undertake?

_____

_____

b. Did Beck begin with a problem statement? Summarize the problem in two to three sentences.

_____

_____

c. Did Beck provide a statement of purpose? What was the purpose?

_____

_____

d. How many different databases did Beck search? Were the searches of electronic databases? Were any manual methods used in the search?

_____

_____

e. What key words were used in the search?

_____

_____

f. Did Beck restrict her search to English-language reports?

_____

_____

g. How many citations were initially identified by the search?

_____

_____

Copyright © 2006. Lippincott Williams & Wilkins. *Study Guide to Accompany Essentials of Nursing Research*, by Denise F. Polit and Cheryl Tatano Beck.

h. How many studies were used in the review?

_____

_____

i. In which countries were the studies conducted?

_____

_____

j. Were the studies included in the review qualitative, quantitative, or both?

_____

_____

QUESTIONS FOR DISCUSSION

a. Did Beck do an adequate job of explaining the problem and the study purpose?

_____

_____

b. Did Beck appear to do a thorough job in her search for relevant studies?

_____

_____

c. The studies included spanned almost 2 decades and were from several different countries. Comment on this.

_____

_____

Copyright © 2006. Lippincott Williams & Wilkins. *Study Guide to Accompany Essentials of Nursing Research*, by Denise F. Polit and Cheryl Tatano Beck.

ACROSS

2. Rhymes with Internet and data set

4. A method of integrating prior findings statistically

7. A report written by researchers who conducted a study is a _____ source in a research review.

8. Used to organize content when writing an extensive literature review

9. A type of search for specific words in text fields of bibliographic records

12. When searching the literature, one often begins by identifying ____ words.

13. In a statistical integration of prior findings, the study itself is the ____ of analysis.

14. The most important bibliographic resource for nurses

Copyright © 2006. Lippincott Williams & Wilkins. *Study Guide to Accompany Essentials of Nursing Research*, by Denise F. Polit and Cheryl Tatano Beck.

15. In summarizing the literature, it is important to point out what _____ there are in the research literature that suggest the need for further research.

20. Computerized literature searches are usually done _____.

21. The MEDLINE database can be accessed for free through the _____MED service.

22. Research literature reviews contain few (if any) clinical _____.

DOWN

1. Literature searches are usually done with the assistance of bibliographic _____bases.

2. A very important bibliographic tool for health care professionals

3. Reviewers covering an extensive literature base often organize their materials in a _____.

4. A tool through which computer software translates topics into appropriate subject terms for a computerized literature search

5. Descriptions of studies prepared by someone other than the investigators are _____ sources (abbr.).

6. Integration of qualitative findings can occur through a meta_____.

9. A resource for finding recent studies is Sigma _____Tau International's Registry of Nursing Research on the Internet.

10. A commercial vendor of bibliographic databases

11. Literature searches can be done with the assistance of a librarian or _____ (without aid) using widely available bibliographic resources.

15. An up-front literature review may not be undertaken by researchers doing a study within the _____ tradition (acronym).

16. Literature reviews are often done to help researchers identify a suitable _____ to investigate (abbr.).

17. Computerized literature searches using _____ databases have replaced manual search methods (abbr.)

18. (Review!) The ethical principle of *beneficence* encompasses the maxim: Above all _____ harm.

19. In doing a computerized search, the number of "_____" can be quite large unless restrictions are placed on the search.

Copyright © 2006. Lippincott Williams & Wilkins. *Study Guide to Accompany Essentials of Nursing Research*, by Denise F. Polit and Cheryl Tatano Beck.

CHAPTER 8

Examining the Conceptual/ Theoretical Basis of a Study

■ A. Matching Exercises

1. *Match each statement from Set B with one of the phrases in Set A. Indicate the letter corresponding to your response next to each of the statements in Set B.*

SET A

a. Classic theory

b. Conceptual framework/model

c. Schematic model

d. Neither a, b, nor c

e. a, b, and c

SET B	**RESPONSES**
1. Makes minimal use of language	_____
2. Uses concepts as building blocks	_____
3. Is essential in the conduct of good research	_____
4. Can be used as a basis for generating hypotheses	_____
5. Can be proved through empirical testing	_____
6. Indicates a system of propositions that assert relationships among variables	_____
7. Consists of interrelated concepts organized in a rational scheme but does not specify formal relationships among the concepts	_____
8. Exists in nature and is awaiting scientific discovery	_____

2. *Match each model from Set B with one of the theorists in Set A. Indicate the letter corresponding to your response next to each of the statements in Set B.*

SET A

a. Orem

b. Pender

Copyright © 2006. Lippincott Williams & Wilkins. *Study Guide to Accompany Essentials of Nursing Research*, by Denise F. Polit and Cheryl Tatano Beck.

c. Roy

d. Becker

e. Rogers

f. Lazarus-Folkman

g. Mishel

h. Azjen

SET B   **RESPONSES**

1. Adaptation Model   _____

2. Health Belief Model   _____

3. Uncertainty in Illness Theory   _____

4. Model of Self-Care   _____

5. Theory of Stress and Coping   _____

6. Health Promotion Model   _____

7. Theory of Planned Behavior   _____

8. Science of Unitary Human Beings   _____

■ B. Completion Exercises

Write the words or phrases that correctly complete the sentences below.

1. Theories are not found by scientists; they are _____.

2. Deductions from theories are referred to as _____.

3. A(n) _____ is the conceptual underpinnings of a study.

4. Most of the conceptualizations of nursing practice would be called _____.

5. Schematic models attempt to represent reality with a minimal use of _____.

6. The four central concepts of conceptual models in nursing are _____,
   _____, _____, and _____.

7. The basic intellectual process underlying theory development is _____.

8. The acronym HPM stands for the _____.

9. Theoretical frameworks from nonnursing disciplines are sometimes referred to as
   _____, but if they have been found to be productive they may be
   called _____.

Copyright © 2006. Lippincott Williams & Wilkins. *Study Guide to Accompany Essentials of Nursing Research,* by Denise F. Polit and Cheryl Tatano Beck.

10. Many qualitative researchers seek to develop a(n) _____

theory, a conceptualization of a phenomenon rooted in the researcher's observations.

■ C. Study Questions

1. Complete the crossword puzzle at the end of the chapter, which uses terms and concepts presented in Chapter 8. (Puzzles may be removed for easier viewing.)

2. Read some recent issues of a nursing research journal. Identify at least two different theories cited by nurse researchers in these research reports.

_____

_____

_____

_____

3. Choose one of the conceptual frameworks of nursing described in this chapter. Develop a research hypothesis based on this framework.

_____

_____

_____

_____

4. Select one of the research questions/problems listed below. Could the selected problem be developed within one of the nursing frameworks discussed in this chapter? Defend your answer.

a. How do men cope with a diagnosis of prostate cancer?

_____

_____

b. What are the factors contributing to perceptions of fatigue among patients with congestive heart failure?

_____

_____

Copyright © 2006. Lippincott Williams & Wilkins. *Study Guide to Accompany Essentials of Nursing Research*, by Denise F. Polit and Cheryl Tatano Beck.

c. What effect does the presence of the father in the delivery room have on the mother's satisfaction with the childbirth experience?

_____

_____

d. The purpose of the study is to explore why some women fail to perform breast self-examination regularly.

_____

_____

e. What are the factors that lead to poorer health among low-income children than higher-income children?

_____

_____

■ D. Application Exercises

1. Read the abstract and introduction of the report by Loeb ("Older Men's Health") in Appendix C. Then answer the following questions:

QUESTIONS OF FACT

a. Does Loeb's study involve a conceptual or theoretical framework? What is it called?

_____

_____

b. Is this framework one of the models of nursing cited in the textbook? Is it related to one of those models?

_____

_____

c. Does the report include a schematic model?

_____

_____

d. What are the key concepts in the model?

_____

_____

Copyright © 2006. Lippincott Williams & Wilkins. *Study Guide to Accompany Essentials of Nursing Research*, by Denise F. Polit and Cheryl Tatano Beck.

e. According to the model, what factors *directly* affect the exercise of self-care agency?

_____

_____

f. According to the model, what factors *directly* affect health outcomes? What factors *indirectly* affect health outcomes?

_____

_____

g. Based on information in the abstract, did the study include a measure of a variable within the "Health-promoting self-care" construct block of the model (Figure 1)?

_____

_____

h. Did the report present conceptual definitions of key concepts?

_____

_____

i. Did the report explicitly present hypotheses deduced from the model?

_____

_____

QUESTIONS FOR DISCUSSION

a. Do the research problem and hypotheses (if any) naturally flow from the framework? Does the link between the problem and the framework seem contrived?

_____

_____

b. Do you think any aspects of the research would have been different without the framework?

_____

_____

c. Could the study have been undertaken using Pender's Health Promotion Model as its framework (see Figure 8-1 in the textbook)? Why or why not?

_____

_____

Copyright © 2006. Lippincott Williams & Wilkins. *Study Guide to Accompany Essentials of Nursing Research,* by Denise F. Polit and Cheryl Tatano Beck.

d. Would you describe this study as a model-testing inquiry, or do you think the model was used more as an organizing framework?

_____

_____

2. Read the introduction and "background" section of the report by Bent ("Empowerment Process") in Appendix D. Then answer the following questions:

QUESTIONS OF FACT

a. Does Bent's study involve a conceptual or theoretical framework? What is it called?

_____

_____

b. Is this framework one of the models of nursing cited in the textbook? Is it related to one of those models?

_____

_____

c. Does the report include a schematic model?

_____

_____

d. What are the key concepts in the framework?

_____

_____

e. Would the framework described in this report best be described as *ideational* or *materialistic*?

_____

_____

f. Did the report present conceptual definitions of key concepts?

_____

_____

g. Did the report explicitly present hypotheses deduced from the framework?

_____

_____

Copyright © 2006. Lippincott Williams & Wilkins. *Study Guide to Accompany Essentials of Nursing Research*, by Denise F. Polit and Cheryl Tatano Beck.

QUESTIONS FOR DISCUSSION

 a. Does the research problem naturally flow from the framework? Does the link between the problem and the framework seem contrived?

 _____

 _____

 b. Do you think any aspects of the research would have been different without the framework?

 _____

 _____

 c. Would you describe this study as a model-testing inquiry, or do you think the model was used more as an organizing framework?

 _____

 _____

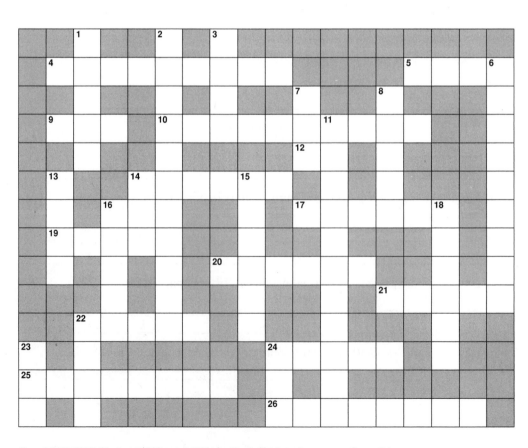

Copyright © 2006. Lippincott Williams & Wilkins. *Study Guide to Accompany Essentials of Nursing Research*, by Denise F. Polit and Cheryl Tatano Beck.

ACROSS

4. The conceptual underpinnings of a study

5. The originator of the Health Promotion Model (abbr.)

9. One of the four elements in conceptual models of nursing (abbr.)

10. Abstractions assembled because of their relevance to a core theme form a _____ model.

12. Psychiatric nurse researchers sometimes obtain funding from an institute within the National Institutes of Health (NIH) with the acronym NI _____.

14. A theory that focuses on a piece of human experience is sometimes called _____-range.

16. Another term for a schematic model is conceptual _____.

17. The originator of the Science of Unitary Human Beings

19. Roy devised the _____ Theory (abbr.).

20. The originator of the Theory of Uncertainty in Illness

21. The originator of the Theory of Human Becoming

22. A schematic _____ is a mechanism for representing concepts with a minimal use of words.

24. The relationship between theory and research has been described as _____ (abbr.), with mutual benefits

25. A theory from another discipline, used to guide nursing inquiry

26. A model of nursing involving what people do on their own behalf to maintain health and well-being

DOWN

1. A theory aimed at explaining large segments of behavior or other phenomena

2. A theory that thoroughly accounts for or describes a phenomenon

3. The social psychologist Bandura originated Social _____ Theory (abbr.).

6. As classically defined, theories consist of concepts arranged in a logically interrelated _____ system.

7. The acronym for Pender's model

8. A theory that focuses on a single piece of human experience is sometimes called middle-_____.

11. If a study is based on a theory, its framework is called the _____ framework.

Copyright © 2006. Lippincott Williams & Wilkins. *Study Guide to Accompany Essentials of Nursing Research*, by Denise F. Polit and Cheryl Tatano Beck.

13. Mathematic equations that express relationships among variables are _____ models (abbr.).

14. A schematic model is also called a conceptual _____.

15. The originator of the Conservation Model of nursing

16. Another name for a grand theory is a _____ theory.

18. A theory originally from another discipline used productively by nurse researchers

22. The originator of the Model of Self-Care (backwards!)

23. The acronym for Becker's model of health behavior

24. Theories are built inductively from observations, which are often obtained in disciplined _____ (abbr.).

Copyright © 2006. Lippincott Williams & Wilkins. *Study Guide to Accompany Essentials of Nursing Research*, by Denise F. Polit and Cheryl Tatano Beck.

PART 3

Designs for Nursing Research

CHAPTER 9

Scrutinizing Quantitative Research Design

■ A. Matching Exercises

1. *Match each research question from Set B with one (or more) of the phrases from Set A that indicates a potential reason for using a nonexperimental design. Indicate the letter(s) corresponding to your response next to each statement in Set B.*

SET A

a. Independent variable cannot be manipulated

b. Possible ethical constraints on manipulation

c. Practical constraints on manipulation

d. No constraints on manipulation

SET B   **RESPONSES**

1. Does the use of certain tampons cause toxic shock syndrome?   _____

2. Does heroin use among pregnant women affect Apgar scores of infants?   _____

3. Is the age of a hemodialysis patient related to the incidence of the disequilibrium syndrome?   _____

4. What body positions aid respiratory function?   _____

5. Does the ingestion of saccharin cause cancer in humans?   _____

6. Does a nurse's attitude toward the elderly affect his or her choice of a clinical specialty?   _____

7. Does the use of touch by nursing staff affect patient morale?   _____

8. Does a nurse's gender affect his or her salary and rate of promotion?   _____

9. Does extreme athletic exertion in young women cause amenorrhea?   _____

10. Does assertiveness training affect a psychiatric nurse's job performance?   _____

Copyright © 2006. Lippincott Williams & Wilkins. *Study Guide to Accompany Essentials of Nursing Research*, by Denise F. Polit and Cheryl Tatano Beck.

■ B. Completion Exercises

Write the words or phrases that correctly complete the sentences below.

1. Researchers generally design their studies to include one or more types of _____ _____ to make their results more interpretable.

2. In an experiment, the researcher manipulates the _____ variable.

3. The manipulation that the researcher introduces is referred to as the experimental _____.

4. Randomization is performed so that groups will be formed without _____.

5. Another term for randomization is _____.

6. When data are gathered before the institution of a treatment, the initial data gathering is referred to as the _____.

7. When more than one independent variable is being simultaneously manipulated by the researcher, the design is referred to as a(n) _____.

8. Each factor in an experimental design must have two or more _____.

9. When neither the subjects nor the individuals collecting data know in which group a subject is participating, the procedures are called _____.

10. Subjects are used as their own controls in a(n) _____ design.

11. A primary objective of a true experiment is to enable the researcher to infer _____ _____.

12. When a true experimental design is not used, the control group is usually referred to as the _____ group.

13. A research design that involves manipulation but lacks the control of a quasi-experiment is referred to as a(n)_____ design.

14. A quasi-experimental design that involves repeated observations over time is referred to as a(n) _____ design.

15. The difficulty with a nonequivalent control group design is that the experimental and comparison groups cannot be assumed to be _____ before the intervention.

16. When no variable is manipulated in a study, the research is called _____.

17. *Ex post facto* research is also referred to as _____ research.

Copyright © 2006. Lippincott Williams & Wilkins. *Study Guide to Accompany Essentials of Nursing Research,* by Denise F. Polit and Cheryl Tatano Beck.

18. In *ex post facto* research, the investigator does not have control over the _____ _____ variable.

19. Correlation does not prove _____.

20. A prospective design is more rigorous in elucidating casual relationships than a(n) _____ design.

21. A retrospective design that involves a comparison of a group with a specified disease or condition with another group without the disease or condition is called a(n) _____ design.

22. When data are collected at more than one point in time, the design is referred to as

_____.

23. Longitudinal studies conducted to determine the long-term outcome of some condition or intervention are called _____.

24. The environment should be controlled by the researcher insofar as possible by maximizing _____ in the research conditions.

25. The specifications of an experimental treatment are often referred to as the _____.

26. Using the principle of homogeneity to control extraneous variables is easy but limits the _____ of the findings.

27. Control over extraneous variables is required for the _____ _____ validity of the study.

28. The most persistent threat to the internal validity of studies arises from preexisting differences between groups, or the _____ threat.

29. Changes that occur as the result of time passing rather than as a result of the treatment represent the threat of _____.

30. Events concurrent with the institution of a treatment that can affect the dependent variable constitute the threat of _____.

31. An inadequate sampling plan can affect the _____ validity of a study.

32. Inadequate power can affect the _____ validity of a study.

■ C. Study Questions

1. Complete the crossword puzzle at the end of the chapter, which uses terms and concepts presented in Chapter 9. (Puzzles may be removed for easier viewing.)

Copyright © 2006. Lippincott Williams & Wilkins. *Study Guide to Accompany Essentials of Nursing Research*, by Denise F. Polit and Cheryl Tatano Beck.

2. Indicate which of the following variables *inherently* can or cannot be manipulated by a researcher.* Assume that ethical constraints are not an issue.

a. Age at onset of obesity

_____

_____

b. Amount of auditory stimulation

_____

_____

c. Number of cigarettes smoked

_____

_____

d. Infant's birth weight

_____

_____

e. Blood type

_____

_____

f. Preoperative anxiety

_____

_____

g. Type of nursing curriculum

_____

_____

h. Attitudes toward evidence-based practice.

_____

_____

_____

*Remember that *manipulation* does not refer to whether or not the variable can be *affected* by a researcher; it refers to the researcher's ability to randomly assign individuals to different levels of the variable or to different groups.

Copyright © 2006. Lippincott Williams & Wilkins. *Study Guide to Accompany Essentials of Nursing Research*, by Denise F. Polit and Cheryl Tatano Beck.

    i. Nurses' shift assignments

_____

_____

    j. Type of birth control method used

_____

_____

    k. Mother–infant bonding

_____

_____

    l. Use of atrioventricular shunt versus atrioventricular fistula

_____

_____

    m. Fluid intake

_____

_____

    n. Morale of dying patients' family members

_____

_____

    o. Nurses' fringe benefits

_____

_____

3. Refer to the 10 hypotheses in Exercises C.3 and C.4 of Chapter 6. Indicate below whether these hypotheses could be tested using an experimental/quasi-experimental approach, a nonexperimental approach, or both.

	EXPERIMENTAL/QUASI-EXPERIMENTAL	NONEXPERIMENTAL	BOTH
3a.	_____	_____	_____
3b.	_____	_____	_____
3c.	_____	_____	_____
3d.	_____	_____	_____
3e.	_____	_____	_____

Copyright © 2006. Lippincott Williams & Wilkins. *Study Guide to Accompany Essentials of Nursing Research*, by Denise F. Polit and Cheryl Tatano Beck.

	EXPERIMENTAL/QUASI-EXPERIMENTAL	NONEXPERIMENTAL	BOTH
4a.	_____	_____	_____
4b.	_____	_____	_____
4c.	_____	_____	_____
4d.	_____	_____	_____
4e.	_____	_____	_____

4. In the following study, the researchers conducted a double-blind experiment. Review the design for this study, and comment on the appropriateness of the double-blind procedures. What biases were the researchers trying to avoid? Do you think they were successful?

   Bale, S., Tebbie, N., & Price, P. (2004). A topical metronidazole gel used to treat malodorous wounds. *British Journal of Nursing, 13*(11), S4–S11.

   _____

   _____

   _____

   _____

5. Suppose that you are studying the effects of range-of-motion exercises on radical mastectomy patients. You start your experiment with 50 experimental subjects and 50 control subjects. Your intervention requires the experimental subjects to come for daily sessions over a 2-week period, while control subjects come only once at the end of 2 weeks. Your final group sizes are 40 for the experimental group and 49 for the control group. The results of your study indicate that the experimental group did better in raising the arm of the affected side above head level. What effects, if any, do you think the subject attrition might have on the internal validity of your study?

   _____

   _____

   _____

   _____

■ D. Application Exercises

1. Read the method section of the report by Gibbins and colleagues ("Procedural Pain") in Appendix A. Then answer the following questions:

Copyright © 2006. Lippincott Williams & Wilkins. *Study Guide to Accompany Essentials of Nursing Research,* by Denise F. Polit and Cheryl Tatano Beck.

QUESTIONS OF FACT

a. Is the design for this study experimental, quasi-experimental, preexperimental, or nonexperimental?

_____

_____

b. What were the independent and dependent variables in this study?

_____

_____

c. Was randomization used? If yes, what method was used to assign subjects to groups?

_____

_____

d. What is the specific name of the research design used in this study?

_____

_____

e. Is the overall design a within-subjects or between-subjects design?

_____

_____

f. Which of the methods of research control described in this chapter were used to control extraneous variables?

_____

_____

g. What extraneous variables were controlled?

_____

_____

h. Could this study be described as double-blind?

_____

_____

i. Was there any attrition in this study?

_____

_____

Copyright © 2006. Lippincott Williams & Wilkins. *Study Guide to Accompany Essentials of Nursing Research,* by Denise F. Polit and Cheryl Tatano Beck.

j. Would this study be described as longitudinal?

_____

_____

k. Is there evidence that constancy of conditions was implemented?

_____

_____

l. Were group treatments as distinct as possible to maximize power? If not, why not?

_____

_____

QUESTIONS FOR DISCUSSION

a. Is this study strong in internal validity? What, if any, are the threats to the internal validity of this study?

_____

_____

b. Is this study strong in external validity? What, if any, are the threats to the external validity of this study?

_____

_____

c. Does this study seem strong in terms of statistical conclusion validity? How could statistical conclusion validity have been strengthened?

_____

_____

2. Read the method section of the report by Loeb ("Older Men's Health") in Appendix C. Then answer the following questions:

QUESTIONS OF FACT

a. Is the design for this study experimental, quasi-experimental, preexperimental, or nonexperimental?

_____

_____

Copyright © 2006. Lippincott Williams & Wilkins. *Study Guide to Accompany Essentials of Nursing Research*, by Denise F. Polit and Cheryl Tatano Beck.

b. What were the independent and dependent variables in this study?

_____

_____

c. Was randomization used? If yes, what method was used to assign subjects to groups?

_____

_____

d. What is the specific name of the research design used in this study?

_____

_____

e. Which of the methods of research control described in this chapter were used to control extraneous variables?

_____

_____

f. What extraneous variables were controlled?

_____

_____

g. Could this study be described as double-blind?

_____

_____

h. Was there any attrition in this study?

_____

_____

i. Would this study be described as longitudinal?

_____

_____

j. Is there evidence that constancy of conditions was implemented?

_____

_____

Copyright © 2006. Lippincott Williams & Wilkins. *Study Guide to Accompany Essentials of Nursing Research*, by Denise F. Polit and Cheryl Tatano Beck.

QUESTIONS FOR DISCUSSION

a. Is this study strong in internal validity? What, if any, are the threats to the internal validity of this study?

_____

_____

b. Is this study strong in external validity? What, if any, are the threats to the external validity of this study?

_____

_____

ACROSS

1. Good research design in quantitative studies involves four aspects of this
4. A design in which the same subjects are exposed to two or more conditions, in random order
6. The loss of subjects from a study over time (abbr.)
9. A threat to internal validity stemming from preexisting group differences
12. In a factorial design, each independent variable is called a _____.
14. A design involving an intervention and certain controls, but not randomization (acronym)
15. The allocation of subjects to groups by chance (acronym)
17. A design in which the independent variable is not manipulated (acronym)
18. In a crossover design, each subject acts as his or her own _____
19. A threat to internal validity stemming from differential loss of subjects from groups
22. A design in which data about presumed causes are collected prior to data about presumed effects (abbr.)
24. The counterfactual in most experimental studies is called the control _____.
25. In a _____d study, different samples from a population are studied over time.
28. Nightingale's first name (first two letters)
29. A type of validity: The degree to which it can be inferred that the independent variable affected the dependent variable (abbr.).
31. The name for the effect on the dependent variable caused by subjects' awareness of being in a study
32. The opposite of out
33. One method of controlling extraneous variables is called analysis of _____.
34. The type of validity referring to the generalizability of results
35. The number of groups in a crossover design
36. Data are collected at a single point in time in a cross-_____ study.

Copyright © 2006. Lippincott Williams & Wilkins. *Study Guide to Accompany Essentials of Nursing Research*, by Denise F. Polit and Cheryl Tatano Beck.

DOWN

2. A posttest-only design involves collecting data only _____ the intervention.

3. A quasi-experimental design involving collection of data multiple times over an extended period (acronym)

4. A nonexperimental design involving the comparison of a case and a matched counterpart

5. A true experiment involves assignment of subjects to groups or conditions at _____.

7. A type of longitudinal study that gathers data from the same people at multiple points in time

8. A research design that involves an intervention but lacks control over extraneous factors is _____experimental.

10. A study designed to collect data over an extended period

11. Another name for an *ex post facto* study (abbr.)

13. An experimental design that collects data once is a posttest-_____ design.

16. An experimental design that collects data prior to the intervention is a before–_____ design.

20. The pairing of subjects in different groups as a method of controlling extraneous variables

21. Designs involving comparisons of different people are _____-subjects designs (abbr.).

23. Statistical _____r involves the ability of the design to detect true relationships among variables.

26. A study designed so that neither subjects nor agents know who got the intervention is _____-blind.

27. One internal validity problem is the history _____.

28. Retrospective studies are a form of *ex post* _____ research.

30. The same subjects are studied under different conditions in a wi _____-subjects design.

32. In an experimental study, the manipulated variable (acronym)

Copyright © 2006. Lippincott Williams & Wilkins. *Study Guide to Accompany Essentials of Nursing Research*, by Denise F. Polit and Cheryl Tatano Beck.

CHAPTER 10

Understanding Qualitative Research Design

■ A. Matching Exercises

1. *Match each descriptive statement from Set B with one of the research traditions from Set A. Indicate the letter corresponding to your response next to each item in Set B.*

SET A

a. Ethnography

b. Phenomenology

c. Grounded theory

d. Ethnography, phenomenology, and grounded theory

SET B   **RESPONSES**

1. Is rooted in a philosophical tradition developed by Husserl and Heidegger   _____

2. Studies both broadly defined cultures and more narrowly defined ones   _____

3. Gathers qualitative data to address questions of interest   _____

4. Is an approach to the study of social processes and social structures   _____

5. Is concerned with the lived experiences of humans   _____

6. Strives to achieve an emic perspective on the members of a group   _____

7. Is closely related to a research tradition called hermeneutics   _____

8. Uses a procedure referred to as constant comparison   _____

9. Stems from a discipline other than nursing   _____

10. Developed by the sociologists Glaser and Strauss   _____

Copyright © 2006. Lippincott Williams & Wilkins. *Study Guide to Accompany Essentials of Nursing Research*, by Denise F. Polit and Cheryl Tatano Beck.

■ B. Completion Exercises

Write the words or phrases that correctly complete the sentences below.

1. The design for a qualitative study is often called a(n) _____ design.

2. Qualitative researchers are often adept at performing many diverse tasks and are sometimes referred to as _____.

3. The disciplinary roots of ethnography are _____; of ethology are _____; and of ethnomethodology are _____.

4. Ethnographic research focuses on human _____.

5. An ethnographic study of a Peruvian village would be called a(n) _____, while an ethnographic study of a ward in a psychiatric hospital would be called a(n) _____.

6. The concept _____ is frequently used by ethnographers to describe the researcher's significant role in interpreting a culture.

7. Phenomenological research focuses on the _____ _____ of phenomena as experienced by people.

8. Phenomenologists study the various aspects of the lived experience including lived space or _____; lived body or _____; lived time or _____; and lived human relation or _____.

9. Bracketing can be enhanced by keeping detailed notes in a(n) _____ _____ journal.

10. Interpretive phenomenology is referred to as _____.

11. The primary purpose of _____ is to generate comprehensive explanations of phenomena that are grounded in reality.

12. In a grounded theory study, the technique referred to as _____ _____ is used to compare new data with previously collected data to identify commonalities and refine categories.

13. Substantive grounded theory can serve as a springboard for _____, _____ which is a higher level of theory.

14. _____ is the systematic collection, evaluation, and synthesis of data relating to past occurrences.

Copyright © 2006. Lippincott Williams & Wilkins. *Study Guide to Accompany Essentials of Nursing Research*, by Denise F. Polit and Cheryl Tatano Beck.

15. Research conducted within the framework known as _____ is action oriented, designed to transform social groups and inspire enlightened self-knowledge.

16. In _____, researchers work closely with participants, often oppressed or vulnerable groups, to produce action for improvements.

■ C. Study Questions

1. Complete the crossword puzzle at the end of the chapter, which uses terms and concepts presented in Chapter 10. (Puzzles may be removed for easier viewing.)

2. For each of the research questions below, indicate what type of qualitative research tradition would likely guide the inquiry.

   a. What is the social psychological process experienced by couples experiencing infertility?

   _____

   _____

   b. How does the culture of a suicide survivors' self-help group contribute to the grieving process?

   _____

   _____

   c. What are the power dynamics that arise in conversations between nurses and bed-ridden nursing home patients?

   _____

   _____

   d. What is the lived experience of the spousal caretaker of an Alzheimer patient?

   _____

   _____

3. Skim the two studies listed below, which are examples of ethnographic and phenomenological studies. What were the central phenomena under investigation? Compare and contrast the methods used in these two studies (e.g., how were data collected? How many study participants were there? To what extent did the design unfold while the researchers were in the field?)

   Ethonographic Study: Tutton, E., & Seers, K. (2004). Comfort on a ward for older people. *Journal of Advanced Nursing, 46,* 380–389.

Copyright © 2006. Lippincott Williams & Wilkins. *Study Guide to Accompany Essentials of Nursing Research,* by Denise F. Polit and Cheryl Tatano Beck.

Phenomenological Study: Enriquez, M., Lackey, N. R., O'Connor, M. C., & McKinsey, D. S. (2004). Successful adherence after multiple HIV treatments. *Journal of Advanced Nursing, 45,* 438–446.

_____

_____

_____

_____

_____

4. Skim the following participatory action research study and comment on the roles of participants and researchers: Choudhry, U. K., Jandu, S., Mahal, J., Singh, R., Sohi-Pabla, H., & Mutta, B. (2002). Health promotion and participatory action research with South Asian women. *Journal of Nursing Scholarship, 34,* 75–81.

_____

_____

_____

_____

_____

■ D. Application Exercises

1. Read the method section of the report by Rew ("Homeless Youth") in Appendix B. Then answer the following questions:

QUESTIONS OF FACT

a. In which tradition was this study based?

_____

_____

b. Which specific approach was used—that of Glaser and Strauss, or that or Strauss and Corbin?

_____

_____

c. What is the central phenomenon under study?

_____

_____

Copyright © 2006. Lippincott Williams & Wilkins. *Study Guide to Accompany Essentials of Nursing Research,* by Denise F. Polit and Cheryl Tatano Beck.

d. Was the study longitudinal?

_____

_____

e. What was the setting for this research?

_____

_____

f. Did the report indicate or suggest that constant comparison was used?

_____

_____

g. Is the research question congruent with a qualitative approach and with the specific research tradition (i.e., is the domain of inquiry for the study congruent with the domain encompassed by the tradition)?

_____

_____

QUESTIONS FOR DISCUSSION

a. How well is the research design described in the report? Are design decisions explained and justified?

_____

_____

b. Does it appear that Rew made all design decisions up-front, or did the design emerge during data collection, allowing her to capitalize on early information?

_____

_____

c. Were there any elements of the design or methods that appear to be more appropriate for a qualitative tradition other than the one Rew identified as the underlying tradition?

_____

_____

2. Read the method section of the report by Bent ("Empowerment Process") in Appendix D. Then answer the following questions:

Copyright © 2006. Lippincott Williams & Wilkins. _Study Guide to Accompany Essentials of Nursing Research,_ by Denise F. Polit and Cheryl Tatano Beck.

QUESTIONS OF FACT

a. In which tradition was this study based?

_____

_____

b. What is the central phenomenon under study?

_____

_____

c. Is this an example of insider research?

_____

_____

d. Is there evidence of "bricolage" in this study?

_____

_____

e. Was the study longitudinal?

_____

_____

f. What was the setting for this research?

_____

_____

g. Is the research question congruent with a qualitative approach and with the specific research tradition (i.e., is the domain of inquiry for the study congruent with the domain encompassed by the tradition)?

_____

_____

QUESTIONS FOR DISCUSSION

a. How well is the research design described? Are design decisions explained and justified?

_____

_____

Copyright © 2006. Lippincott Williams & Wilkins. *Study Guide to Accompany Essentials of Nursing Research*, by Denise F. Polit and Cheryl Tatano Beck.

b. Does it appear that the researcher made all design decisions up-front, or did the design emerge during data collection, allowing the researcher to capitalize on early information?

_____

_____

c. Does the report convince you that Bent was able to achieve an emic perspective?

_____

_____

d. Was the study undertaken with an ideological perspective? If so, is there evidence that ideological methods and goals were achieved? (e.g., was there evidence of full collaboration between the researcher and participants? Did the research have the power to be transformative, or is there evidence that a transformative process occurred?)

_____

_____

ACROSS

5. Leininger's phrase for research at the interface between culture and nursing

7. The type of phenomenology that includes the step of bracketing (abbr.)

10. The type of ethnographic research wherein researchers study their own culture or subculture

11. Research that focuses on gender domination

14. A type of psychological research that studies the environment's influence on behavior (abbr.)

15. One of the two originators of grounded theory

18. A type of action research (acronym)

20. Knowledge that is so embedded in a culture that people do not talk about it

21. A type of phenomenology sometimes called hermeneutics (abbr.)

22. The perspective that is the outsider's view

25. Qualitative researchers' efforts to derive information from a wide array of sources

26. Traditional qualitative research does not adopt a strong political point of view or _____ perspective (abbr.).

27. Qualitative research design decisions typically unfold while researchers are in the _____.

29. Qualitative research that is not done within any specific tradition is typically called _____ (abbr.).

31. Qualitative research design is typically a(n) _____ design.

DOWN

1. A qualitative tradition concerned with social processes and social structures (acronym)

2. Experimental design is held in high regard in quantitative research, but in qualitative research a flexible design is the _____ standard.

3. Phenomenologists study _____ experiences.

4. One aspect of experience that phenomenologists study is spatiality or _____ (acronym).

5. The perspective that is the insider's view.

Copyright © 2006. Lippincott Williams & Wilkins. *Study Guide to Accompany Essentials of Nursing Research*, by Denise F. Polit and Cheryl Tatano Beck.

6. The systematic collection and analysis of materials relating to the past is _____ research.

7. The type of analysis designed to understand the rules and structure of conversations.

8. The nurse researcher who worked with an originator of grounded theory to develop an alternative approach

9. A type of phenomenology focusing on the *meaning* of experiences (abbr.)

12. The second step in descriptive phenomenology is to in_____.

13. A phenomenological question is: What is the _____ of this phenomenon? (abbr.)

16. Research that involves a critique of society is based on _____ theory.

17. The biology of human behavior

19. An aspect of experience that phenomenologists study is relationality or lived human _____ (backwards!).

20. An approach to classifying qualitative research design is according to qualitative _____ (abbr.).

23. Qualitative researchers often maintain a _____ journal to record their own presuppositions and biases (abbr.).

24. Qualitative designs are _____ experimental.

25. The phenomenological concept _____-in-the-world acknowledges people's physical ties to their world.

28. Another term for insider ethnography (abbr.)

30. A procedure in grounded theory research used to develop and refine categories (acronym)

Copyright © 2006. Lippincott Williams & Wilkins. *Study Guide to Accompany Essentials of Nursing Research*, by Denise F. Polit and Cheryl Tatano Beck.

CHAPTER 11

Examining Specific Types of Research

■ A. Matching Exercises

1. *Match each feature from Set B with one (or more) of the phrases from Set A that indicates a type of quantitative research. Indicate the letter(s) corresponding to your response next to each statement in Set B.*

SET A

a. Clinical trial

b. Evaluation research

c. Methodologic research

d. Survey research

e. Outcomes research

f. Secondary analysis

SET B   **RESPONSES**

1. Can involve an experimental design   _____

2. Cost-benefit analyses are one type.   _____

3. Examines the global effectiveness of nursing services   _____

4. Data are always from self-reports.   _____

5. The aim is to develop better instruments and procedures for substantive research.   _____

6. Often designed in a series of phases (typically four)   _____

7. Includes process analyses   _____

8. Benefits from controls over extraneous variables   _____

9. The most well-known type is the RCT.   _____

10. Avoids time-consuming and costly research steps   _____

Copyright © 2006. Lippincott Williams & Wilkins. *Study Guide to Accompany Essentials of Nursing Research,* by Denise F. Polit and Cheryl Tatano Beck.

■ B. Completion Exercises

Write the words or phrases that correctly complete the sentences below.

1. Phase III trials may be referred to as _____.

2. Phase II clinical trials are often considered a _____ of an intervention.

3. A _____ analysis provides descriptive information about how a policy or program actually works in practice.

4. Impact analyses use an experimental or quasi-experimental design to determine a program's _____ effects.

5. A _____ is used to determine whether monetary benefits of an intervention outweigh costs.

6. _____ is undertaken to document the effectiveness of health care services.

7. Methodologic research is so named because it is research conducted for the purpose of developing or refining research _____.

8. In surveys, _____ interviews are less expensive than in-person interviews.

9. When a researcher analyzes data as a secondary analysis and either aggregates or disaggregates the data differently than in the original research, we say that there has been a change in the _____.

10. A _____ is an in-depth investigation of a single entity or small number of entitites.

11. Qualitative and quantitative data may, for some research problems, be _____ _____ in that they "mutually supply each other's lack."

12. A major advantage of integrating different approaches in a single study is potential enhancements to the study's _____.

13. A frequent application of multimethod studies is in the development of research

_____.

14. In studies of the effects of complex interventions, qualitative data may be useful in addressing the _____ question.

Copyright © 2006. Lippincott Williams & Wilkins. *Study Guide to Accompany Essentials of Nursing Research*, by Denise F. Polit and Cheryl Tatano Beck.

■ C. Study Questions

1. Complete the crossword puzzle at the end of the chapter, which uses terms and concepts presented in Chapter 11. (Puzzles may be removed for easier viewing.)

2. In what ways are impact analyses and phase III clinical trials similar and different?

_____

_____

_____

_____

3. Suppose you were interested in studying the research questions below by conducting a survey. For each, indicate whether you would recommend using a personal interview, a telephone interview, or a self-administered questionnaire to collect the data. What is your rationale?

   a. What are the coping strategies and behaviors of newly widowed individuals?

   _____

   _____

   b. Are the rural elderly more socially isolated than the urban elderly?

   _____

   _____

   c. What type of nursing communications do presurgical patients find most helpful?

   _____

   _____

   d. What is the relationship between a teenager's health-risk appraisal and his or her risk-taking behavior (e.g., smoking, unprotected sex, drug use, etc.)?

   _____

   _____

   e. What are the health-promoting activities pursued by inner-city single mothers?

   _____

   _____

   f. How is employment of parents affected by the health problems or disability of a child?

   _____

   _____

Copyright © 2006. Lippincott Williams & Wilkins. *Study Guide to Accompany Essentials of Nursing Research*, by Denise F. Polit and Cheryl Tatano Beck.

4. Read one of the studies below, in which quantitative data were gathered and analyzed to address a research question. Suggest ways in which the collection of qualitative data might have enriched the study, strengthened its validity, or enhanced its interpretability.

   Collins, E., Langbein, W. E., Dilan-Koetje, J., Bammert, C., Hanson, K., Reda, D., et al. (2004). Effects of exercise training on aerobic capacity and quality of life in individuals with heart failure. *Heart & Lung, 33,* 154–161.

   McCurry, S. M., Gibbons, L. E., Logsdon, R. G, & Teri. L. (2004). Anxiety and nighttime behavioral disturbances: Awakenings in patients with Alzheimer's disease. *Journal of Gerontological Nursing, 30,* 12–20.

   Vallerand, A. H., Riley-Doucet, C., Hasenau, S., & Templin, T. (2004). Improving cancer pain management by homecare nurses. *Oncology Nursing Forum, 31,* 809–816.

5. Below is a brief description of a mixed method study, followed by a critique. Do you agree with this critique? Can you add other comments regarding the study design?

   Fictitious Study. Tacy conducted a study designed to examine the emotional well-being of women who had a mastectomy. Tacy wanted to develop an in-depth understanding of the emotional experiences of women as they recovered from their surgery, including the process by which they handled their fears, their concerns about their sexuality, their levels of anxiety and depression, their methods of coping, and their social supports.

   Tacy's basic study design was a qualitative field study, loosely within a grounded theory tradition. She gathered information from a sample of 26 women, primarily by means of in-depth interviews with the women on two occasions. The first interviews were scheduled within 1 month after the surgery. Follow-up interviews were conducted about 12 months after the surgery. Several of the women in the sample participated in a support group, and Tacy attended and made observations at several of those meetings. Additionally, Tacy decided to interview the "significant other" (usually the women's husbands) of most of the women, when it became clear that the women's emotional well-being was linked to the manner in which the significant other was reacting to the surgery.

   In addition to the rich, in-depth information she gathered, Tacy wanted to be able to better interpret the emotional status of the women. Therefore, at both the original and follow-up interviews with the women, she administered a psychological scale known as the Center for Epidemiological Studies Depression Scale (CES-D), a quantitative measure that has scores that can range from 0 to 60. This scale has been widely used in community populations, and has cut-off scores designating when a person is at risk of clinical depression (i.e., a score of 16 and above).

   Tacy's qualitative analysis showed that the basic process underlying psychological recovery from the mastectomy was something she labeled "Gaining by Losing," a process that involved heightened self-awareness and self-respect after an initial period of despair and self-pity. The process also involved, for some, a strengthening of personal relationships with significant others, whereas for others, it resulted in the birth of awareness of fundamental deficiencies in their relationships. The quantitative findings confirmed that a very high percentage of women were at risk of being

Copyright © 2006. Lippincott Williams & Wilkins. *Study Guide to Accompany Essentials of Nursing Research,* by Denise F. Polit and Cheryl Tatano Beck.

depressed at 1 month after the mastectomy, but at 12 months, the average level of depression was actually modestly lower than in the general population of women.

Critique.   In her study, Tacy embedded a quantitative measure into her fieldwork in an interesting manner. The bulk of data were qualitative—in-depth interviews and in-depth observations. However, she also opted to include a well-known measure of depression, which provided her with an important context for interpreting her data. A major advantage of using the CES-D is that this scale has known characteristics in the general population, and therefore provided a built-in "comparison group."

Tacy used a flexible design that allowed her to use her initial data to guide her inquiry. For example, she decided to conduct in-depth interviews with significant others when she learned their importance to the women's process of emotional recovery. Tacy did do some advance planning, however, that provided loose guidance. For example, although her questioning undoubtedly evolved while in the field, she had the foresight to realize that to capture a process as it evolved, she would need to collect data longitudinally. She also made the up-front decision to use the CES-D to supplement the in-depth interviews.

In this study, the findings from the qualitative and quantitative portions of the study were complementary. Both portions of the study confirmed that the women initially had emotional "losses," but eventually they recovered and "gained" in terms of their emotional well-being and their self-awareness. This example illustrates how the validity of study findings can be enhanced by the blending of qualitative and quantitative data. If the qualitative data alone had been gathered, Tacy might not have gotten a good handle on the degree to which the women had actually "recovered" (vis à vis women who had never had a mastectomy). Conversely, if she had collected only the CES-D data, she would have had no insights into the process by which the recovery occurred.

■ D. Application Exercises

1. Which of the studies in the appendices of this Study Guide could be considered a case study?

2. Which of the studies in the appendices of this Study Guide could be considered survey research?

3. Read the first few sections (the sections before "results") of the report by Egan and her colleagues ("Nursing-Based Case Management") in Appendix E. Then answer the following questions:

QUESTIONS OF FACT

a. Was this study a clinical trial? If yes, what phase trial would this most likely be?

_____

_____

Copyright © 2006. Lippincott Williams & Wilkins. *Study Guide to Accompany Essentials of Nursing Research*, by Denise F. Polit and Cheryl Tatano Beck.

b. Was this study an evaluation? If yes, what type (process analysis, etc.)?

_____

_____

c. Was this outcomes research?

_____

_____

d. Was this study a secondary analysis?

_____

_____

e. Was this study a survey?

_____

_____

f. Was this a case study?

_____

_____

g. Was this study an example of methodologic research?

_____

_____

h. What is the basic research design for this study (i.e., experimental, nonexperimental, etc.)?

_____

_____

i. Was this a mixed method study? If yes, what strategy of integration was used?

_____

_____

QUESTIONS FOR DISCUSSION

a. Is this study strong in internal validity? What, if any, are the threats to the internal validity of this study?

_____

_____

Copyright © 2006. Lippincott Williams & Wilkins. *Study Guide to Accompany Essentials of Nursing Research*, by Denise F. Polit and Cheryl Tatano Beck.

b. Does this study seem strong in terms of statistical conclusion validity? How could statistical conclusion validity have been strengthened?

_____

_____

c. Comment on the adequacy and appropriateness of the use of various types of data in this study. How, if at all, did data of different types strengthen the study? How could the design have been strengthened further?

_____

_____

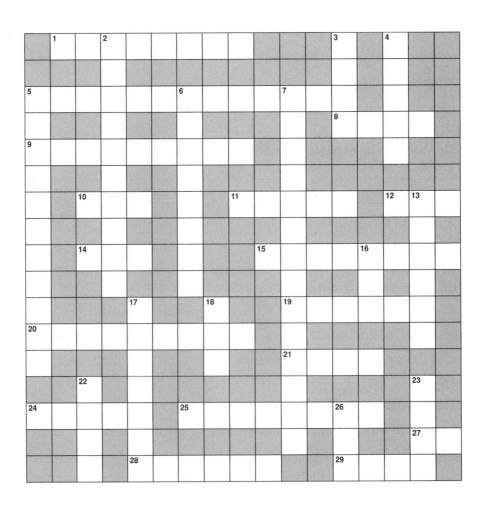

ACROSS

1. Interviews that are done in person
5. A study to refine and test the effectiveness of a clinical intervention
8. Another term for interviews done in person is _____ to _____.
9. An analysis of data done with an existing data set
10. The phase of a trial that is an RCT
11. Surveys can be done by distributing these (abbr.).
12. One goal of mixed-method research is to generate and test _____ (abbr.) in a single study.
14. An impact analysis provides information about _____ effects.
15. This type of research focuses on improving research strategies (abbr.).
19. An alternative to in-person interviews is interviews by _____ (abbr.).
20. A method of collecting self-report data orally
21. A phase II trial can be a pilot _____.
24. In clinical trials, an RCT is the third _____.
25. Research to document the effectiveness of health care services
27. The final phase of a clinical trial
28. A Gallup poll is one of these.
29. The type of evaluation most like a phase III clinical trial is an im _____ analysis.

DOWN

2. A phase III clinical trial is _____.
3. Data collected by asking people questions is via _____ reports.
4. A _____ box question may emerge in interpreting the effects of a complex intervention.
5. An evaluation of the monetary effects of an intervention
6. One type of evaluation is an outcome _____.
7. An analysis that describes the process of putting a new intervention into place
13. The most ambitious application of multimethod research involves the building of _____ (backwards!).

Copyright © 2006. Lippincott Williams & Wilkins. *Study Guide to Accompany Essentials of Nursing Research,* by Denise F. Polit and Cheryl Tatano Beck.

16. The number of entities in a typical case study

17. Another name for an implementation analysis

18. Sometimes surveys can be administered over the _____ (abbr.).

22. An in-depth study of a single entity is a _____ study.

23. Sometimes a secondary analysis involves a change in the _____ of analysis.

26. An RCT involves the use of a(n) _____ design (abbr.).

Copyright © 2006. Lippincott Williams & Wilkins. *Study Guide to Accompany Essentials of Nursing Research,* by Denise F. Polit and Cheryl Tatano Beck.

CHAPTER 12

Examining Sampling Plans

■ A. Matching Exercises

1. Match each statement relating to sampling for quantitative studies from Set B with one of the phrases from Set A. Indicate the letter corresponding to your response next to each of the statements in Set B.

SET A

a. Probability sampling

b. Nonprobability sampling

c. Both probability and nonprobability sampling

d. Neither probability nor nonprobability sampling

SET B   **RESPONSES**

1. Includes systematic sampling   _____

2. Allows an estimation of the magnitude of sampling error   _____

3. Guarantees a representative sample   _____

4. Includes quota sampling   _____

5. Requires a sample size of at least 100 subjects   _____

6. Elements are selected by nonrandom methods   _____

7. Can be used with entire populations or with selected strata
   from the populations   _____

8. Used to select populations   _____

9. Elements have an equal chance of being selected   _____

10. Is required when the population is homogeneous   _____

2. Match each type of sampling approach from Set B with one of the phrases from Set A. Indicate the letter corresponding to your response next to each of the statements in Set B.

SET A

a. Sampling approach for quantitative studies

b. Sampling approach for qualitative studies

Copyright © 2006. Lippincott Williams & Wilkins. *Study Guide to Accompany Essentials of Nursing Research*, by Denise F. Polit and Cheryl Tatano Beck.

c. Sampling approach for either quantitative or qualitative studies

d. Sampling approach for neither quantitative nor qualitative studies

SET B   **RESPONSES**

1. Typical case sampling   _____

2. Purposive sampling   _____

3. Cluster sampling   _____

4. Deviant case sampling   _____

5. Homogeneous sampling   _____

6. Snowball sampling   _____

7. Stratified random sampling   _____

8. Quota sampling   _____

9. Power sampling   _____

10. Theoretical sampling   _____

■ B. Completion Exercises

Write the words or phrases that correctly complete the sentences below.

1. A(n)_____ is a subset of the units that comprise the population.

2. The main criterion for evaluating a sample in a quantitative study is its _____
   _____ of the population being studied.

3. A sample in a quantitative study would be considered _____
   if it systematically overrepresented or underrepresented a segment of the population.

4. If a population is completely _____
   with respect to key attributes, then any sample is as good as any other.

5. Another term used for purposive sample is _____ sample.

6. Quota samples are essentially convenience samples from selected _____
   _____ of the population.

7. Another term for convenience sampling in a quantitative context is _____
   _____ sampling; in a qualitative context, the term
   _____ sampling is sometimes used for convenience sampling.

Copyright © 2006. Lippincott Williams & Wilkins. *Study Guide to Accompany Essentials of Nursing Research*, by Denise F. Polit and Cheryl Tatano Beck.

8. The most basic type of probability sampling is referred to as _____
_____ sampling.

9. The actual list from which a random sample is drawn is referred to as the _____
_____.

10. When disproportionate sampling is used, an adjustment procedure known as _____
_____ is normally used to estimate population values.

11. Another term used to refer to cluster sampling is _____
_____ sampling.

12. In systematic samples, the distance between selected elements is referred to as the
_____.

13. Differences between population values and sample values are referred to as _____
_____.

14. If a quantitative researcher has confidence in his or her sampling design, the results
of a study can reasonably be generalized to the _____
_____ population.

15. As the size of a sample _____
_____, the probability of drawing a deviant sample diminishes.

16. If a researcher wanted to draw a systematic sample of 100 from a population of
3000, the sampling interval would be _____.

17. In a qualitative study, sampling decisions are often guided by the potential a data
source has to be _____ -rich.

18. In _____ sampling, the qualitative researcher deliberately
reduces variation, while in _____ sampling, the researcher
purposefully selects cases with a wide range of variation on dimensions of interest.

19. _____ sampling
involves selecting study participants to highlight the average situation.

20. Grounded theory researchers rely on _____
sampling to include informants who can best contribute to the emerging theory.

21. Toward the end of the study, qualitative researchers often seek to sample _____
_____ or _____ cases.

Copyright © 2006. Lippincott Williams & Wilkins. *Study Guide to Accompany Essentials of Nursing Research*, by Denise F. Polit and Cheryl Tatano Beck.

22. Ethnographers have conversations with dozens of people but often rely on a very small

    sample of _____ to act as guides to the culture.

■ C. Study Questions

1. Complete the crossword puzzle at end of the chapter, which uses terms and concepts presented in Chapter 12. (Puzzles may be removed for easier viewing.)

2. For each of the following target populations, identify an accessible population (accessible to *you*) that might be used in a study.

Target Population   *Accessible Population*

   a. All teenagers diagnosed as having   _____

      scoliosis   _____

   b. All nursing home residents over the   _____

      age of 70 years   _____

   c. All rape victims in metropolitan areas _____

   d. All individuals with blood type   _____

      O positive   _____

3. Identify the type of quantitative sampling design used in the following examples:

   a. One hundred inmates randomly sampled from a random selection of five federal

      penitentiaries _____

   b. All the nurses participating in a continuing education seminar _____

      _____

   c. Every 20th patient admitted to the emergency room between January and June

      _____

   d. The first 20 male and the first 20 female patients admitted to the hospital with

      hypothermia _____

   e. A sample of 250 members randomly selected from a roster of American Nurses

      Association members _____

4. Nurse A is planning to study the effects of maternal stress, maternal depression, maternal age, and family economic resources on a child's socioemotional development among both intact and mother-headed families. Nurse B is planning to study body position on patients' respiratory functioning. Describe the kinds of samples that the

Copyright © 2006. Lippincott Williams & Wilkins. *Study Guide to Accompany Essentials of Nursing Research*, by Denise F. Polit and Cheryl Tatano Beck.

two nurses would need to use. Which nurse would need the larger sample? Defend your answer.

_____

_____

_____

_____

_____

5. Suppose a qualitative researcher wanted to study the life quality of cancer survivors. Suggest what the researcher might do to obtain a maximum variation sample, a typical case sample, a homogeneous sample, and an extreme case sample.

_____

_____

_____

_____

_____

■ D. Application Exercises

1. Which of the studies in the appendices of this Study Guide (if any) used a probability sample?

_____

_____

2. Which of the studies in the appendices of this Study Guide used quota sampling?

_____

_____

3. Read the method section of the report by Loeb ("Older Men's Health") in Appendix C. Then answer the following questions:

QUESTIONS OF FACT

a. What was the target population of Loeb's study? How would you describe the accessible population?

_____

_____

Copyright © 2006. Lippincott Williams & Wilkins. *Study Guide to Accompany Essentials of Nursing Research*, by Denise F. Polit and Cheryl Tatano Beck.

b. What were the eligibility criteria for the study?

_____

_____

c. Was Loeb's sampling method probability or nonprobability? What specific sampling method was used?

_____

_____

d. How were study participants recruited?

_____

_____

e. What efforts did Loeb make to ensure a diverse (and hence more representative) sample?

_____

_____

f. What was the sample size that Loeb achieved?

_____

_____

g. Was a power analysis used to determine sample size needs? If yes, what number of subjects did the power analysis estimate as the minimum needed number?

_____

_____

QUESTIONS FOR DISCUSSION

a. Comment on the adequacy of Loeb's sampling plan and recruitment strategy. How representative was the sample of the target population? What types of sampling biases might be of special concern?

_____

_____

b. Do you think Loeb's sample size was adequate? Why or why not?

_____

_____

Copyright © 2006. Lippincott Williams & Wilkins. *Study Guide to Accompany Essentials of Nursing Research*, by Denise F. Polit and Cheryl Tatano Beck.

4. Read the method section of the report by Rew ("Homeless Youth") in Appendix B. Then answer the following questions:

QUESTIONS OF FACT

a. What were the eligibility criteria for this study?

_____

_____

b. How were study participants recruited?

_____

_____

c. What type of sampling approach was used?

_____

_____

d. How many study participants comprised the sample?

_____

_____

e. Was data saturation achieved?

_____

_____

f. Did Rew's sampling strategy include confirming and disconfirming cases?

_____

_____

QUESTIONS FOR DISCUSSION

a. Comment on the adequacy of Rew's sampling plan and recruitment strategy for achieving the goals of a grounded theory study.

_____

_____

b. Do you think Rew's sample size was adequate? Why or why not?

_____

_____

Copyright © 2006. Lippincott Williams & Wilkins. *Study Guide to Accompany Essentials of Nursing Research*, by Denise F. Polit and Cheryl Tatano Beck.

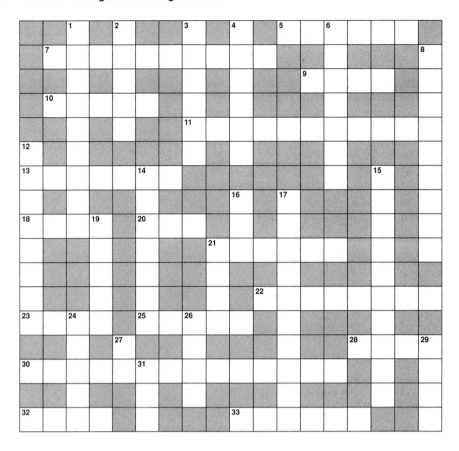

ACROSS

5. The population that is available to a researcher (abbr.)

7. An aggregate set of individuals or objects with specified characteristics

9. Another name for purposive sampling (abbr.)

10. Another name for cluster sampling is _____ -stage.

11. The type of sampling preferred by grounded theory researchers

13. The most basic unit of a population

18. A sampling approach in which participants are hand-picked because of known attributes (abbr.)

20. Ethnographers might begin sampling using a big ___ approach.

21. A sampling approach in which every kth element is selected (abbr.)

22. The specific attributes of a population are designated through eligibility _____ .

Copyright © 2006. Lippincott Williams & Wilkins. *Study Guide to Accompany Essentials of Nursing Research*, by Denise F. Polit and Cheryl Tatano Beck.

23. A qualitative sampling approach in which the most unusual or deviant cases are selected (abbr.)

25. A strong sampling design can enhance the study's value for evidence- _____ practice.

28. A distortion that arises when a sample is not representative of the population is a sampling _____.

30. In quantitative studies, the key criterion for evaluating a sample is whether it is _____ of the population.

32. Criteria designating characteristics a population does *not* have (abbr.)

33. A probability sample involves selection at _____ .

DOWN

1. A term used in qualitative studies in lieu of "convenience" sample

2. Sampling by convenience, but within specified strata

3. Subdivisions of a population

4. The most widely used type of sampling in quantitative research (abbr.)

6. Probability sampling involving successive random selection of smaller units

8. Criteria specifying characteristics that a population must have

12. The rate of participation in a study is the _____ rate.

14. Sampling methods in which not every element of a population has an equal chance of being selected (abbr.)

15. Cases selected in a qualitative study to verify preliminary findings

16. Ethographers rely on a sample of _____ informants.

17. The principle used by qualitative researchers to determine when to stop sampling

19. The analysis used by quantitative researchers to estimate the number of subjects needed

21. The number of participants in a study is the sample _____ .

24. A qualitative sampling approach that yields participants who are "average" (abbr.)

26. A common survey approach is to _____ sample members a questionnaire through the mail.

27. Incorrect values are yielded in a study when there is _____ (acronym).

29. A sampling method involving referrals from other people already in the sample (abbr.)

31. The most basic type of probability sampling (acronym)

Copyright © 2006. Lippincott Williams & Wilkins. *Study Guide to Accompany Essentials of Nursing Research*, by Denise F. Polit and Cheryl Tatano Beck.

PART 4

Data Collection

CHAPTER 13

Scrutinizing Data Collection Methods

■ A. Matching Exercises

1. Match each descriptive statement regarding data collection methods from Set B with one (or more) of the statements from Set A. Indicate the letter(s) corresponding to your response next to each item in Set B.

SET A

a. Self-reports

b. Observations

c. Biophysiologic measures

d. None of the above

SET B   **RESPONSES**

1. Cannot easily be gathered unobtrusively   _____

2. Can be biased by the subject's desire to "look good"   _____

3. Can be used to gather data from infants   _____

4. Is rarely used in qualitative studies   _____

5. Is a good way to obtain information about human *behavior*   _____

6. Can be biased by the researcher's values and beliefs   _____

7. Can be combined with other data collection methods in a single study   _____

8. Can range from highly unstructured to highly structured data   _____

9. Can yield quantitative information   _____

10. Benefits from pretesting   _____

2. Match each descriptive statement regarding self-report methods from Set B with one of the statements from Set A. Indicate the letter corresponding to your response next to each item in Set B.

Copyright © 2006. Lippincott Williams & Wilkins. *Study Guide to Accompany Essentials of Nursing Research*, by Denise F. Polit and Cheryl Tatano Beck.

SET A

a. Interviews

b. Questionnaires

c. Both interviews and questionnaires

d. Neither interviews nor questionnaires

SET B	RESPONSES
1. Can provide respondents the protection of anonymity	_____
2. Can be used with illiterate respondents	_____
3. Can contain both open- and closed-ended questions	_____
4. Is used in grounded theory studies	_____
5. Is the best way to measure human behavior	_____
6. Generally yields high response rates	_____
7. Can control the order in which questions are asked and answered	_____
8. Is generally an inexpensive method of data collection	_____
9. Requires that the purpose of the study be unknown to the study participant	_____
10. Benefits from pretesting	_____
11. Can be used in longitudinal studies	_____
12. Can be distributed by mail	_____

■ B. Completion Exercises

Write the words or phrases that correctly complete the sentences below.

1. The four dimensions along which data collection methods can vary are _____, _____, _____, and _____.

2. _____ is the dimension that could result in distortions on the part of subjects who are engaged in socially unacceptable behavior.

3. The data collection approach that is especially high on objectivity is _____ _____.

4. The major advantage of using existing records is that they are _____ _____.

Copyright © 2006. Lippincott Williams & Wilkins. *Study Guide to Accompany Essentials of Nursing Research*, by Denise F. Polit and Cheryl Tatano Beck.

5. When we want to know what people's attitudes are, we are most likely to use the broad method of _____.

6. Completely unstructured interviews generally begin with a broad, informal question, sometimes referred to as a _____ question.

7. In semistructured interviews, general question areas are normally listed on a(n)

   _____.

8. When a group of respondents is assembled in one place to discuss questions simultaneously, the interview is called a(n) _____.

9. The approach used to question people about key events, decisions, or turning points is referred to as the _____ technique.

10. The _____ method is used to gather information about cognitive processes, such as decision making.

11. A disadvantage of _____ questions is that researchers may inadvertently omit some potentially important response alternatives.

12. Questions that offer only two response options are known as _____

    _____ items.

13. Likert scales consist of a number of statements written in the _____

    _____ form.

14. In Likert scales, positively worded statements are scored in one direction, and the scoring of negatively worded statements is _____.

15. Respondents rate concepts on a series of bipolar adjectives in the _____

    _____ technique.

16. A(n) _____ can be used to measure subjective experiences (e.g., fatigue) along a 100 mm line.

17. The bias introduced when respondents select options at either end of the response continuum is known as _____.

18. In a Q sort, subjects are generally instructed to place cards in _____ or _____ piles.

19. _____ are brief descriptions of individuals or situations to which subjects are asked to react.

Copyright © 2006. Lippincott Williams & Wilkins. *Study Guide to Accompany Essentials of Nursing Research*, by Denise F. Polit and Cheryl Tatano Beck.

20. The major focus of observation in nursing research is human _____ _____.

21. When observers are not hidden or unobtrusive, the biasing effect called _____ _____ may result in behavioral distortions.

22. The technique known as _____ involves the collection of unstructured observational data in which observers play a role in the group or culture being observed.

23. Chronological notes about observers' use of their time are maintained in a(n) _____.

24. In structured observations, the most common procedure is to construct a(n) _____ _____that designates the behaviors or events to be observed.

25. _____ is the method of obtaining representative observations by selecting time periods during which observations will occur.

26. Observers need to be carefully _____ _____ in the use of a structured observational instrument.

27. Biophysiologic measures that are taken directly within a living organism are _____ _____measures.

28. When biophysiologic materials are extracted from people and subjected to analysis, the data are referred to as _____ measures.

■ C. Study Questions

1. Complete the crossword puzzle at the end of the chapter, which uses terms and concepts presented in Chapter 13.(Puzzles may be removed for easier viewing.)

2. Below are several research problems. Indicate what methods of data collection (self-report, observation, biophysiologic measures, records) you might recommend using for each. Defend your response.

   a. How does an elderly patient manage the transition from hospital to home?

   _____

   _____

Copyright © 2006. Lippincott Williams & Wilkins. *Study Guide to Accompany Essentials of Nursing Research*, by Denise F. Polit and Cheryl Tatano Beck.

b. What are the predictors of a suicide attempt?

_____

_____

c. What are the social psychological factors associated with smoking during pregnancy?

_____

_____

d. To what extent and in what manner do nurses interact differently with male and female patients?

_____

_____

e. What are the coping mechanisms of parents whose infants are long-term patients in neonatal intensive care units?

_____

_____

3. For each of the research problems in Question C.2, indicate where on the four dimensions discussed in this chapter (structure, quantifiability, researcher obtrusiveness, and objectivity) the method of data collection would most likely lie.

4. Below are several research problems. Indicate which type of unstructured self-report approach you might recommend using for each. Defend your response.

a. By what process do parents of a handicapped child learn to cope with their child's disability?

_____

_____

b. What are the barriers to preventive health care practices among the urban poor?

_____

_____

c. What stresses does the spouse of a terminally ill patient experience?

_____

_____

Copyright © 2006. Lippincott Williams & Wilkins. *Study Guide to Accompany Essentials of Nursing Research,* by Denise F. Polit and Cheryl Tatano Beck.

d. What type of information does a nurse draw on most heavily in formulating pain management decisions?

_____

_____

e. What are the coping mechanisms and perceived barriers to coping among severely disfigured burn patients?

_____

_____

5. Suppose you were interested in studying the frustrations of patients waiting for treatment in the waiting area of an emergency department. Develop a topic guide for a semistructured interview on this topic.

6. For the study described in Question C.5, develop five closed-ended questions. Compare the nature of the information you would obtain for the research problem described in Question C.5 using the topic guide versus using the closed-ended questions. Which approach would yield more useful information? Defend your response.

7. Identify five constructs of clinical relevance that would be appropriate for measurement using a visual analog scale (VAS).

_____

_____

_____

_____

_____

8. Below are several research questions in which the dependent variable is amenable to observation. For each question, specify whether you think a structured or unstructured approach would be preferable. Justify your response.

a. What is the effect of touch on the crying behavior of hospitalized children? _____

_____

_____

b. What is the effect of increased patient/staff ratios in psychiatric hospitals on interpersonal conflict among patients? _____

_____

_____

Copyright © 2006. Lippincott Williams & Wilkins. *Study Guide to Accompany Essentials of Nursing Research,* by Denise F. Polit and Cheryl Tatano Beck.

c. Are the self-grooming activities of nursing home patients related to the frequency of visits from friends and relatives? _____

_____

_____

d. What is the process by which very-low-birth-weight infants develop the sucking response? _____

_____

_____

e. What type of patient behaviors are most likely to elicit empathic behaviors in nurses? _____

_____

_____

f. Do nurses reinforce passive behaviors among female patients more than among male patients? _____

_____

_____

9. Using procedures described in Chapter 13, suggest ways of collecting data on the following variables: fear of death among the elderly; body image among amputees; reactions to the onset of menarche; anxiety; quality of life; nurses' morale in an emergency room; and dependence among cerebral palsied children.

■ D. Application Exercises

1. Which of the studies in Appendices B (by Rew), C (by Loeb), and E (by Egan et al.) of this Study Guide used the following data collection methods:
   ■ Self-reports
   ■ Observational methods
   ■ Biophysiologic measures

2. Read the method section of the report by Gibbins and coresearchers ("Procedural Pain") in Appendix A—specifically the subsections labeled "outcome measures" and "procedures." Then answer the following questions:

Copyright © 2006. Lippincott Williams & Wilkins. *Study Guide to Accompany Essentials of Nursing Research*, by Denise F. Polit and Cheryl Tatano Beck.

QUESTIONS OF FACT

a. How would you describe the data collection methods of this study in terms of structure, quantifiability, obtrusiveness, and objectivity?

_____

_____

b. Did the researchers develop their own measures, or did they use instruments or scales that had been developed by others?

_____

_____

c. Did this study use any self-report measures? If no, could they have been used to measure key concepts? If yes, what specific types of self-reports were used? How were self-report data recorded? What variables were measured by self-report?

_____

_____

d. Did this study collect any data through observation? If no, could observation have been used to measure key concepts? If yes, what variables were measured through observation? How were data obtained and recorded? What type of sampling was used, if any?

_____

_____

e. Did this study collect any biophysiologic measures? If no, could such measures have been used to capture key concepts? If yes, what variables were measured through biophysiologic methods? Were the measures in vitro or in vivo? How were the measurements made?

_____

_____

f. Were records used in this study? If no, could records have been used to measure key concepts? If yes, what records were used and what variables were captured?

_____

_____

g. Who gathered the data in this study? How were the data collectors trained?

_____

_____

Copyright © 2006. Lippincott Williams & Wilkins. *Study Guide to Accompany Essentials of Nursing Research*, by Denise F. Polit and Cheryl Tatano Beck.

h. Does the report indicate that steps were taken to verify the quality of the data that were gathered?

_____

_____

QUESTIONS FOR DISCUSSION

a. Comment on the adequacy of the data collection approaches used in this study. Did Gibbins and her colleagues operationalize their outcome measures in the best possible manner?

_____

_____

b. Comment on the procedures used to collect data in this study. Were adequate steps taken to ensure the highest possible quality data?

_____

_____

3. Read the research design section of the report by Bent ("Empowerment process") in Appendix D—specifically the subsections labeled "data generation" and "methods." Then answer the following questions:

QUESTIONS OF FACT

a. How would you describe the data collection methods of this study in terms of structure, quantifiability, obtrusiveness, and objectivity?

_____

_____

b. Did this study collect any self-report data? If no, could self-reports have been used? If yes, what concepts were captured by self-reports? What specific types of qualitative self-report methods were used? How were self-report data recorded?

_____

_____

c. Did this study collect any data through observation? If no, could observation have been used? If yes, what concepts were captured through observation? How were data obtained and recorded?

_____

_____

Copyright © 2006. Lippincott Williams & Wilkins. *Study Guide to Accompany Essentials of Nursing Research*, by Denise F. Polit and Cheryl Tatano Beck.

d. Did this study collect any biophysiologic measures? If no, could such measures have been used to capture important concepts? If yes, what variables were measured through biophysiologic methods? Were the measures in vitro or in vivo? How were the measurements made?

_____

_____

e. Were records, documents, or artifacts used in this study? If no, could they have been used? If yes, what records were used and what concepts were captured?

_____

_____

f. Who collected the data in this study? How were the data collectors trained?

_____

_____

g. Does the report indicate that steps were taken to verify the quality of the data that were gathered?

_____

_____

QUESTIONS FOR DISCUSSION

a. Comment on the adequacy of the data collection approaches used in this study. Did Bent fully capture the concepts of interest in the best possible manner?

_____

_____

b. Comment on the procedures used to collect data in this study. Were adequate steps taken to ensure the highest possible quality data?

_____

_____

Copyright © 2006. Lippincott Williams & Wilkins. *Study Guide to Accompany Essentials of Nursing Research,* by Denise F. Polit and Cheryl Tatano Beck.

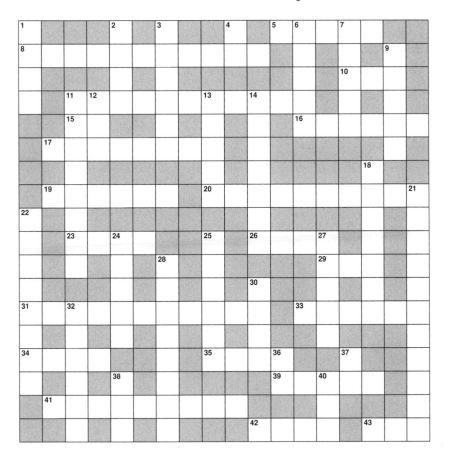

ACROSS

5. A tool that yields a score placing people on a continuum with regard to an attribute

8. A type of observation used in ethnographies and grounded theory studies

10. In unstructured observation, information needs about processes are "_____" questions (backwards!).

11. The type of question most prevalent in mailed questionnaires

15. A type of question that involves placing response alternatives in a systematic order (acronym)

16. Data collection in which specific questions/observations and possible responses/ categories are specified in advance (abbr.)

17. A description of a situation or person designed to elicit study participants' reactions

Copyright © 2006. Lippincott Williams & Wilkins. *Study Guide to Accompany Essentials of Nursing Research*, by Denise F. Polit and Cheryl Tatano Beck.

19. A scaling procedure to measure clinical symptoms is a _____ analog scale.

20. A procedure for gathering data about decision making or problem solving as it unfolds

23. A type of response bias stemming from a tendency to always agree (abbr.)

26. The most widely used method of data collection by nurse researchers is by _____-report.

29. On a summated rating scale, if SD was scored as five, SA would be scored as _____.

31. A method of collecting data by watching behaviors and events

33. _____ research tends to use data collection methods that are low on structure (abbr.)

34. An interview guided by an established list of broad topics is _____ structured.

35. Unstructured interviews are typically _____, sometimes lasting hours.

39. A written guide used in some qualitative studies to ensure that important question areas are covered

41. The type of self-report method that typically yields better-quality data than self-administered questionnaires

42. The sampling approach in observational studies to select periods when observations are made

43. A straight line, typically measuring 100 mm, to measure such concepts as pain and fatigue (acronym)

DOWN

1. The question "What is it like to be a cancer survivor?" is _____-ended.

2. Measures obtained within or on living organisms are in _____.

3. A summated rating scale used to measure agreement or disagreement with statements

4. Extracting biophysiologic material from people yields _____ vitro measures.

6. In Q-sorts, the objects being sorted are _____.

7. Mailed questionnaires tend to have _____ response rates than telephone interviews.

9. In structured observation, a _____ list is used with a category system to record frequencies.

11. The _____ incidents technique involves in-depth exploration of specific events or episodes.

Copyright © 2006. Lippincott Williams & Wilkins. *Study Guide to Accompany Essentials of Nursing Research,* by Denise F. Polit and Cheryl Tatano Beck.

12. Participant observers maintain a record of daily events and conversations in a _____.

13. Observational sampling of integral episodes

14. Study participants may be asked to maintain ongoing records of some aspect of their lives in _____.

18. Sometimes observers prefer to _____ themselves to ensure more naturalistic behavior among those being observed.

21. A type of question with only two response options, such as yes or no

22. The question "What is your gender?" has two _____ alternatives.

24. An approach involving the sorting of statements into different piles along a continuum

25. A bias stemming from people's wanting to "look good" is called a(n) _____ desirability bias.

27. A technique for gathering in-depth information from a group of informants is called a _____ group interview.

28. The bias stemming from distortions of behavior because of the known presence of an observer (abbr.)

30. One advantage of questionnaires is that _____ can be ensured to protect privacy (abbr.).

32. Respondents rate concepts on a series of bipolar rating scales in a _____ differential (abbr.).

36. A broad opening question in an unstructured interview to gain an overview (acronym)

37. A rating scale along the continuum "exhausted" to "energized" is using _____ polar adjectives.

38. The tendency to distort self-report information in characteristic ways is called a response-_____ bias.

40. Structured instruments are almost always subjected to a _____ test before being used in an actual study.

Copyright © 2006. Lippincott Williams & Wilkins. *Study Guide to Accompany Essentials of Nursing Research,* by Denise F. Polit and Cheryl Tatano Beck.

CHAPTER 14

Evaluating Measurements and Data Quality

■ A. Matching Exercises

1. *Match each statement from Set B with one of the phrases from Set A. Indicate the letter corresponding to your response next to each of the statements in Set B.*

SET A

a. Reliability

b. Validity

c. Both reliability and validity

d. Neither reliability nor validity

SET B RESPONSES

1. Is concerned with the accuracy of measures _____

2. The measures must be high on this for the results of a study to be valid. _____

3. If a measure possesses this, then study findings are necessarily sound. _____

4. Can in some cases be estimated by procedures that yield a quantified coefficient _____

5. May in some cases be assessed by scrutinizing the components (items) of the measure _____

6. Is necessarily high when the measure is high on objectivity _____

7. Is concerned with whether the researcher has adequately conceptualized the variables under investigation _____

8. Coefficient alpha is an index for this _____

9. Psychometric assessments evaluate this. _____

10. Is used to establish a cutoff point for screening instruments _____

2. *Match each statement from Set B with one of the phrases from Set A. Indicate the letter corresponding to your response next to each of the statements in Set B.*

Copyright © 2006. Lippincott Williams & Wilkins. *Study Guide to Accompany Essentials of Nursing Research*, by Denise F. Polit and Cheryl Tatano Beck.

SET A

a. Data source triangulation

b. Investigator triangulation

c. Theory triangulation

d. Method triangulation

SET B   **RESPONSES**

1. A researcher studying health beliefs of the rural elderly interviews old people and health care providers in the area.   _____

2. A researcher tests narrative data, collected in interviews with people who attempted suicide, against two alternative explanations of stress and coping.   _____

3. Two researchers independently interview 10 informants in a study of adjustment to a cancer diagnosis and debrief with each other to review what they have learned.   _____

4. A researcher studying school-based clinics observes interactions in the clinics and also conducts in-depth interviews with students.   _____

5. A researcher studying the process of resolving an infertility problem interviews husbands and wives separately.   _____

6. Themes emerging in the field notes of an observer on a psychiatric ward are categorized and labeled independently by the researcher and an assistant.   _____

▪ B. Completion Exercises

Write the words or phrases that correctly complete the sentences below.

1. People are not measured directly; their _____ are measured.

2. _____
_____ communicates how much of an attribute is present in an object.

3. In measurement, numbers are assigned according to specified _____.

4. Obtained scores almost always consist of an error component and a(n) _____
_____ component.

5. From a measurement perspective, response-set biases represent a source of _____
_____.

6. A reliable measure is one that maximizes the _____
_____ component of observed scores.

Copyright © 2006. Lippincott Williams & Wilkins. *Study Guide to Accompany Essentials of Nursing Research*, by Denise F. Polit and Cheryl Tatano Beck.

7. Test–retest reliability focuses on the _____ of a measure.

8. The most widely used index of internal consistency is _____.

9. Procedures that examine the proportion of agreement between two independent judges yield estimates of _____.

10. An instrument that is not reliable cannot be _____.

11. A measure that looks as though it is measuring what it purports to measure is said to have _____ validity.

12. The type of validity that focuses on the representativeness of the measure's subparts is _____ validity.

13. The type of validity that deals with the ability of an instrument to distinguish individuals who differ in terms of some future criterion is _____ validity.

14. The known-groups technique is a method used to evaluate an instrument's _____ validity.

15. A(n) _____ is a process undertaken specifically to assess the reliability and validity of an instrument.

16. _____ is the ability of a screening instrument to correctly identify cases, and _____ is its ability to correctly identify noncases.

17. The four criteria for establishing the trustworthiness of qualitative data are _____, _____, _____, and _____.

18. When qualitative researchers undertake _____ in the field, they have more opportunity to develop trust with informants and to test for possible misinformation.

19. The use of multiple sources of information in a study as a means of verification is known as _____.

20. _____ is the technique of debriefing with informants to evaluate the credibility of the analysis of qualitative data.

21. The criterion of _____ refers to the objectivity or neutrality of qualitative data.

22. In qualitative studies, a(n) _____ of data and documents by an independent reviewer can verify the dependability and neutrality of the data and their interpretation.

Copyright © 2006. Lippincott Williams & Wilkins. *Study Guide to Accompany Essentials of Nursing Research*, by Denise F. Polit and Cheryl Tatano Beck.

■ C. Study Questions

1. Complete the crossword puzzle at the end of the chapter, which uses terms and concepts presented in Chapter 14. (Puzzles may be removed for easier viewing.)

2. The reliability of measures of which of the following attributes would *not* be appropriately assessed using a test–retest procedure with 1 month between administrations. Why?

   a. Attitudes toward abortion:

   _____

   _____

   b. Stress:

   _____

   _____

   c. Achievement motivation:

   _____

   _____

   d. Nursing effectiveness:

   _____

   _____

   e. Depression:

   _____

   _____

3. Comment on the meaning and implications of the following statement: A researcher found that the internal consistency of her 20-item scale measuring attitudes toward nurse-midwives was .74, using the Cronbach alpha formula.

   _____

   _____

   _____

   _____

   _____

Copyright © 2006. Lippincott Williams & Wilkins. *Study Guide to Accompany Essentials of Nursing Research*, by Denise F. Polit and Cheryl Tatano Beck.

4. In the following situation, what might be some of the sources of measurement error?

One hundred nurses who worked in a large metropolitan hospital were asked to complete a 10-item Likert scale designed to measure job satisfaction. The questionnaires were distributed by nursing supervisors at the end of shifts. The staff nurses were asked to complete the forms and return them immediately to their supervisors.

_____

_____

_____

_____

5. Identify what is incorrect about the following statements:

a. "My scale is highly reliable, so it must be valid."

_____

_____

b. "My instrument yielded an internal consistency coefficient of .80, so it must be stable."

_____

_____

c. "The validity coefficient between my scale and a criterion measure was .40; therefore, my scale must be of low validity."

_____

_____

d. "My scale had a reliability coefficient of .80. Therefore, an obtained score of 20 is indicative of a true score of 16."

_____

_____

e. "The validation study proved that my measure has construct validity."

_____

_____

f. "My advisor examined my new measure of dependence in nursing home residents and, based on its content, assured me the measure was valid."

_____

_____

Copyright © 2006. Lippincott Williams & Wilkins. *Study Guide to Accompany Essentials of Nursing Research,* by Denise F. Polit and Cheryl Tatano Beck.

6. Below is a brief description of a fictitious study, followed by a critique. Do you agree with the critique? Can you add other comments relevant to issues discussed in Chapter 14 of the textbook?

Fictitious Study. Kettlewell developed a 12-item Likert scale that measured feelings of loneliness and social isolation among the elderly. Examples of the items include, "I have lots of friends with whom I am close" and "Sometimes days go by without my having a real conversation with anyone." Kettlewell pretested her instrument with 50 men and women aged 65 to 75 years living independently in the community. She estimated the reliability of the scale using internal consistency procedures (Cronbach's alpha), which yielded a reliability coefficient of .61.

Kettlewell took two steps to validate her scale. First, she asked two geriatric nurses to examine the 12 items to assess the scale's content validity. These experts suggested some wording changes on three items and recommended replacing one other. Next, she compared the scale scores of 100 elderly widows and widowers with those of 100 elderly married men and women. Her rationale was that the widowed would probably feel lonelier as a group than the nonwidowed. Her expectation was confirmed. Kettlewell concluded that her scale was reasonably valid and reliable.

Critique. Kettlewell took some reasonable steps in constructing her scale and assessing its quality. For example, it appears that she included a sufficient number of items (12) to yield discriminating scores. She used the Cronbach's alpha approach, which is the best method available for assessing the internal consistency of Likert scales.

The reliability of Kettlewell's scale, however, could and should be improved. The reliability coefficient of .61 suggests that there is considerable measurement error. There are several steps that Kettlewell could take to try to raise the reliability. First, she could make sure that each item on her scale is doing the job it was intended to do. Remember that scales are designed to discriminate among people who possess different amounts of some trait, in this case social isolation. If Kettlewell identifies one or more items for which there is little variability (i.e., most respondents either agree or disagree), then the item should be discarded. It is probably not measuring social isolation if everyone responds the same way. Kettlewell should also consider lengthening the scale. Other things being equal, longer scales are more reliable than shorter ones.

Kettlewell's efforts to validate her scale also deserve comment. Her first step was to consider the content validity of the scale. Having two knowledgeable people examine the scale was a desirable thing to do. Nevertheless, it cannot be said that this activity in itself ensured the validity of the scale. As a second step, Kettlewell used the known-groups technique. The data she obtained provided some useful evidence of the scale's construct validity. After making some of the revisions suggested above to improve the scale's reliability, however, Kettlewell would do well to gather some additional data to support the scale's construct validity. For example, one might suspect that people would feel less socially isolated if they reported having kin living within a 20-mile radius; if they had visited with a friend within a 72-hour period preceding the completion of the scale; and if they were active members of a club, church group, or other social organization. All of these expectations could be tested. If Kettlewell took

Copyright © 2006. Lippincott Williams & Wilkins. *Study Guide to Accompany Essentials of Nursing Research*, by Denise F. Polit and Cheryl Tatano Beck.

these additional steps to establish the reliability and validity of her scale and obtained favorable results, she could be more confident that the quality of her scale was high.

■ D. Application Exercises

1. Read the method section of the report by Loeb ("Older Men's health") in Appendix C—specifically the subsections on the instruments. Then answer the following questions:

QUESTIONS OF FACT

a. Which of the following methods were used to collect data in this study:
   - Self-reports
   - Observation
   - Biophysiologic measures

b. Did the methods used in this study yield quantitative or qualitative data?

_____

_____

c. Were any data collected by interview? By questionnaire? If the former, were the interviews face-to-face or telephone? If the latter, how were the questionnaires distributed?

_____

_____

d. Describe what methods (if any) were reported as having been used to assess the reliability of the following instruments:
   - The demographics instrument
   - Older Men's Health Program and Screening Inventory
   - Health-Promotion Activities of Older Adults Measure
   - Health Self-Determinism Index

_____

_____

e. Describe what methods (if any) were reported as having been used to assess the validity of the following instruments:
   - The demographics instrument
   - Older Men's Health Program and Screening Inventory
   - Health-Promotion Activities of Older Adults Measure
   - Health Self-Determinism Index

_____

_____

Copyright © 2006. Lippincott Williams & Wilkins. *Study Guide to Accompany Essentials of Nursing Research*, by Denise F. Polit and Cheryl Tatano Beck.

f. Did Loeb rely on assessments of quality from other researchers, or did she herself perform any quality assessments?

_____

_____

QUESTIONS FOR DISCUSSION

a. Describe what some of the sources of measurement error might have been in this study.

_____

_____

b. Comment on the quality of the measures that Loeb used in her study. Do you feel confident that they were adequately reliable and valid indicators of the key constructs?

_____

_____

2. Read the method section of the report by Rew ("Homeless Youth") in Appendix B— specifically the subsections labeled "procedure" and "data analysis." Then answer the following questions:

QUESTIONS OF FACT

a. Which of the following methods were used to collect data in this study:

▪ Self-reports
▪ Observation
▪ Biophysiologic measures

b. Did the methods used in this study yield quantitative or qualitative data?

_____

_____

c. Were any data collected by interview? By questionnaire? If the former, were the interviews face-to-face or telephone? If the latter, how were the questionnaires distributed?

_____

_____

Copyright © 2006. Lippincott Williams & Wilkins. _Study Guide to Accompany Essentials of Nursing Research,_ by Denise F. Polit and Cheryl Tatano Beck.

d. Were any of the following methods used to enhance the credibility of the study and its data:

- ■ Prolonged engagement and/or persistent observation
- ■ Triangulation
- ■ Peer debriefing
- ■ Member checks
- ■ Search for disconfirming evidence
- ■ Researcher credibility
- ■ Other methods

_____

_____

e. Describe what methods (if any) were used to enhance the following aspects of the study:

- ■ Dependability
- ■ Confirmability or auditability
- ■ Transferability

_____

_____

QUESTIONS FOR DISCUSSION

a. Discuss the thoroughness with which Rew described her efforts to evaluate the trustworthiness of her data and her overall study.

_____

_____

b. How would you characterize the trustworthiness of this study, based on Rew's documentation?

_____

_____

Copyright © 2006. Lippincott Williams & Wilkins. *Study Guide to Accompany Essentials of Nursing Research*, by Denise F. Polit and Cheryl Tatano Beck.

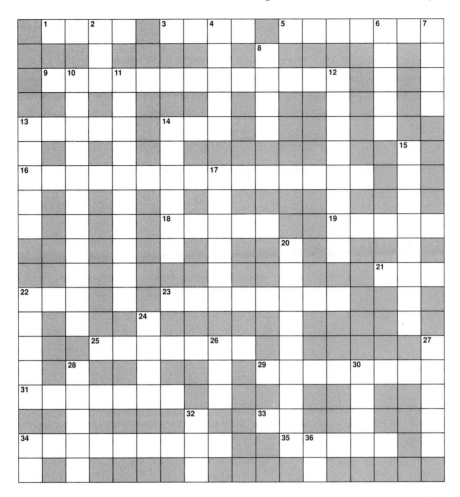

ACROSS

1. The type of validity involving the extent to which a measure "looks" valid

3. The reliability method used to assess stability is _____–retest.

5. The type of validity concerned with adequate representation of all aspects of a concept

9. Use of multiple methods to converge on the truth

13. Measurement involves assigning numbers according to established _____.

14. In screening instruments, the point used to separate "cases" and "noncases" is called the _____ off.

16. Extent to which qualitative findings can be applied to other settings

18. One means of assessing construct validity is through the _____ -groups technique.

Copyright © 2006. LIPPINCOTT WILLIAMS & WILKINS. *Study Guide to Accompany Essentials of Nursing Research*, by Denise F. Polit and Cheryl Tatano Beck.

19. If a measure is unreliable it cannot possibly be _____.

21. Credibility can be enhanced through a thorough search for _____ confirming evidence that challenges preliminary conclusions.

22. One source of measurement error in psychosocial scales is the bias caused by a response _____.

23. The most widely evaluated aspect of reliability is a measure's _____ consistency.

25. To _____ an attribute involves assigning numeric values to designate its quantity.

29. The coefficient alpha index was developed by a psychologist whose last name was _____.

31. The aspect of reliability being evaluated through interobserver methods is _____ (abbr.).

33. The index that is computed to estimate a measure's validity (acronym)

34. Predictive validity and concurrent validity are aspects of _____-related validity.

35. Qualitative researchers evaluate the _____ worthiness of their data and their methods.

DOWN

2. The indicator summarizing assessments of a measure's content validity (acronym)

4. An early method of assessing internal consistency was the _____ half method.

6. The difference between an obtained score and the true score is the _____ of measurement.

7. The score on a measure that would be obtained if the measure were infallible

8. A source of measurement error in scales or tests is _____ sampling.

10. The degree of consistency or accuracy of a measure indicates its _____.

11. A thorough evaluation of an instrument involves a psychometric _____.

12. Refinement of a theory or description through the inclusion of potentially disconfirming cases is a _____ case analysis.

13. When two people independently assign ratings, accuracy is estimated through inter_____ reliability procedures.

14. An important method of assessing credibility involves member _____.

15. Auditability can be enhanced by a(n) _____ trail that documents judgments and choices.

Copyright © 2006. Lippincott Williams & Wilkins. *Study Guide to Accompany Essentials of Nursing Research*, by Denise F. Polit and Cheryl Tatano Beck.

17. An assumption made in measurement is that everything exists in some _____ .

20. The degree to which an instrument is measuring the abstract concept it is supposed to be measuring is _____ validity.

22. If a person got a 29 on a Likert scale, that would be his or her obtained _____ .

24. Interviewing patients *and* family members about a phenomenon is an example of _____ source triangulation.

26. One of the categories of information assembled as part of an audit trail is the _____ data.

27. Transferability is enhanced if researchers use _____ description.

28. A scrutiny of information in a qualitative study to enhance confirmability involves an inquiry _____ .

30. Measurement error can be the result of any systematic _____ in an instrument.

32. In measurement, _____ are assigned to objects (common acronym).

34. The most widely used index of internal consistency (acronym)

36. The index that is computed as an estimate of a measure's reliability (acronym)

Copyright © 2006. Lippincott Williams & Wilkins. *Study Guide to Accompany Essentials of Nursing Research*, by Denise F. Polit and Cheryl Tatano Beck.

PART 5

Data Analysis

CHAPTER 15

Analyzing Quantitative Data

■ A. Matching Exercises

1. *Match each variable in Set B with the level of measurement from Set A that captures the highest possible level for that variable. Indicate the letter corresponding to your response next to each variable in Set B.*

SET A

a. Nominal scale

b. Ordinal scale

c. Interval scale

d. Ratio scale

SET B   **RESPONSES**

1. Hours spent in labor before childbirth   _____

2. Religious affiliation   _____

3. Time to first postoperative voiding   _____

4. Responses to a single Likert scale item   _____

5. Temperature on the centigrade scale   _____

6. Nursing specialty area   _____

7. Status on the following scale: in poor health; in fair health; in good health; in excellent health   _____

8. Pulse rate   _____

9. Score on a 25-item Likert scale   _____

10. Highest college degree attained (bachelor's, master's, doctorate)   _____

11. Apgar scores   _____

12. Membership in the American Nurses Association   _____

2. *Match each phrase from Set B with one of the phrases from Set A. Indicate the letter corresponding to your response next to each of the statements in Set B.*

SET A

a. Measure(s) of central tendency

b. Measure(s) of variability

c. Measure(s) of neither central tendency nor variability

d. Measure(s) of both central tendency and variability

SET B	RESPONSES
1. The range	_____
2. In lay terms, an average	_____
3. A percentage	_____
4. Descriptor(s) of a distribution of scores	_____
5. Descriptor(s) of how heterogeneous a set of values is	_____
6. The standard deviation	_____
7. The mode	_____
8. The median	_____
9. A normal distribution	_____
10. The mean	_____

3. *Match each statement from Set B with one of the phrases in Set A. Indicate the letter corresponding to your response next to each of the statements in Set B.*

SET A

a. Parametric test

b. Nonparametric test

c. Neither parametric nor nonparametric tests

d. Both parametric and nonparametric tests

SET B	RESPONSES
1. The chi-squared test	_____
2. Paired *t*-test	_____
3. Researcher establishes the risk of type I errors	_____
4. Used when a score distribution is markedly non-normal	_____
5. Offers proof that the null hypothesis is either true or false	_____
6. Assumes the dependent variable is measured on an interval or ratio scale	_____

Copyright © 2006. Lippincott Williams & Wilkins. *Study Guide to Accompany Essentials of Nursing Research*, by Denise F. Polit and Cheryl Tatano Beck.

7. Uses sample data to estimate population values   _____

8. ANOVA   _____

9. Computed statistics are compared to tabled values based on theoretical distributions   _____

10. Pearson's *r*   _____

■ B. Completion Exercises

Write the words or phrases that correctly complete the sentences below.

1. Nominal measurement involves a simple _____ _____ of objects according to some criterion.

2. Rank-order questions are an example of _____ measures.

3. With ratio-level measures there is a real, rational _____.

4. Unlike ordinal measures, interval measures involve _____ _____ between points on the scale.

5. A descriptive index (e.g., percentage) from a population is called a(n) _____ _____.

6. A(n) _____ is a systematic arrangement of quantitative data from lowest to highest values.

7. A _____ _____ is a common way of presenting frequency information in graphic form.

8. A distribution is described as _____ _____ if the two halves are mirror images of each other.

9. A distribution is described as _____ skewed if its longer tail points to the left.

10. A distribution that has only one peak is said to be _____.

11. Many human characteristics, such as height and intelligence, are distributed to approximate a(n) _____.

12. Measures that summarize the typical value in a distribution are known as measures of _____.

Copyright © 2006. Lippincott Williams & Wilkins. *Study Guide to Accompany Essentials of Nursing Research,* by Denise F. Polit and Cheryl Tatano Beck.

13. Measures of _____

    are concerned with how spread out the data are.

14. When scores are not very spread out (i.e., dispersed over a wide range of values), the

    sample is said to be _____ with respect to that variable.

15. The most widely used measure of variability is the _____.

16. Descriptive statistics for two variables examined simultaneously are called _____

    _____.

17. Relationships are described as _____

    _____ if high values on one variable are associated with low values on a second.

18. The most commonly used correlation index is _____.

19. Researchers using quantitative analysis apply _____

    to draw conclusions about a population based on information from a sample.

20. Sampling distributions of means have a _____ distribution.

21. The desired degree of risk of making a(n) _____

    _____ error is established by the researcher.

22. Tests that involve the estimation of parameters are referred to as _____

    _____ tests.

23. The most commonly used _____

    _____ are the .05 and .01 levels.

24. Using $\alpha = .01$ rather than $\alpha = .05$ *increases* the risk of committing a _____

    _____ error.

25. In a(n) _____, differences in means for two groups are tested, while in

    a(n) _____, differences in means for three or more groups are tested.

26. The statistic computed in an analysis of variance is the _____ statistic.

27. When both the independent and dependent variables are nominal measures, the test

    statistic usually calculated is the _____.

28. The analysis that would be used to predict patients' postoperative fatigue levels on

    the basis of three preoperative characteristics would be _____.

29. The square of _____ indicates the proportion

    of variance accounted for in a dependent variable by several independent variables.

Copyright © 2006. Lippincott Williams & Wilkins. *Study Guide to Accompany Essentials of Nursing Research*, by Denise F. Polit and Cheryl Tatano Beck.

30. Multiple correlation coefficients can range in value from _____ to

_____ .

31. ANCOVA is shorthand for _____ .

32. In ANCOVA, an extraneous variable being controlled is referred to as a(n) _____

_____ .

33. The multivariate procedure used to reduce a large number of variables to a smaller

set of unified dimensions is _____ .

34. If the independent variables were gender, age, and cigarette smoking status and the

dependent variable was lung cancer status (ever had/never had), the analysis could

either be _____ or _____ .

35. The procedure known as _____

transforms the probability of an event occurring into an odds ratio.

36. Two procedures that are used in causal modeling are _____ and

_____ .

■ C. Study Questions

1. Complete the crossword puzzle at the end of the chapter, which uses terms and concepts
   presented in Chapter 15. (Puzzles may be removed for easier viewing.)

2. Name five physiologic measures that yield ratio-level measurements.

   a. _____

   b. _____

   c. _____

   d. _____

   e. _____

3. Prepare a frequency distribution and frequency polygon for the set of scores below,
   which represent the ages of 30 women receiving hormone replacement therapy:

   47 50 51 50 48 51 50 51 49 51
   54 49 49 53 51 52 51 52 50 53
   49 51 52 51 50 55 48 54 53 52

Copyright © 2006. Lippincott Williams & Wilkins. *Study Guide to Accompany Essentials of Nursing Research,* by Denise F. Polit and Cheryl Tatano Beck.

Describe the resulting distribution in terms of its symmetry and modality (i.e., whether it is unimodal or multimodal).

_____

_____

_____

_____

_____

4. Calculate the mean, median, and mode for the following pulse rates:

    78 84 69 98 102 72 87 75 79 84 88 84 83 71 73

    Mean: _____

    Median: _____

    Mode: _____

5. A group of nurse researchers measured the amount of time (in minutes) spent in recreational activities by a sample of 200 hospitalized paraplegic patients. They compared male and female patients as well as those aged 50 and younger versus those over 50 years old. The four group means (50 subjects per group) were as follows

Age	Male	Female
≤50 years	98.2	70.1
>50	50.8	68.3

A two-way ANOVA yielded the following results:

	F	df	p
Gender	3.61	1, 196	NS
Age group	5.87	1, 196	$<.05$
Gender × Age group	6.96	1, 196	$<.01$

Interpret the meaning of these results.

_____

_____

_____

_____

_____

Copyright © 2006. Lippincott Williams & Wilkins. *Study Guide to Accompany Essentials of Nursing Research*, by Denise F. Polit and Cheryl Tatano Beck.

6. The correlation between the number of days absent per year and annual salary in a sample of 100 nurses was found to be − .23 ($p < .05$). What does this result mean?

_____

_____

_____

_____

_____

7. Indicate which statistical tests you would use to analyze data for the following variables:

a. Variable 1 is psychiatric patients' gender; variable 2 is whether or not the patient has attempted suicide in the past 6 months.

_____

_____

b. Variable 1 is the participation versus nonparticipation of patients with a pulmonary embolus in a special treatment program; variable 2 is the pH of the patients' arterial blood gases.

_____

_____

c. Variable 1 is serum creatinine concentration levels; variable 2 is daily urine output.

_____

_____

d. Variable 1 is patients' marital status (married versus divorced/separated/widowed versus never married); variable 2 is the patients' degree of self-reported depression (measured on a 30-item depression scale).

_____

_____

8. In the following examples, which multivariate procedure is most appropriate for analyzing the data?

a. A researcher is testing the effect of verbal expressiveness, self-esteem, age, and the availability of family supports among a group of recently discharged psychiatric patients on recidivism (i.e., whether they will be readmitted within 12 months after discharge).

_____

_____

Copyright © 2006. Lippincott Williams & Wilkins. *Study Guide to Accompany Essentials of Nursing Research*, by Denise F. Polit and Cheryl Tatano Beck.

b. A researcher is comparing scores on a coping scale of recently widowed and divorced individuals, controlling for their age.

_____

_____

c. A researcher wants to test the effects of two drug treatments and two dosages of each drug on blood pressure, and the pH and PO_2 levels of arterial blood gases.

_____

_____

d. A researcher wants to predict hospital staff absentee rates (number of days absent) based on staff rank, shift, number of years with the hospital, and marital status.

_____

_____

■ D. Application Exercises

1. Read the results section of the report by Gibbins and colleagues ("Procedural Pain") in Appendix A. Then answer the following questions:

QUESTIONS OF FACT

a. Referring to Table 1, answer the following questions:

■ Which three descriptive statistics are presented in this table?

_____

_____

■ Does the table present any inferential statistics?

_____

_____

■ Which variable described in the table is a nominal-level variable?

_____

_____

■ Are there any ordinal-level variables in the table?

_____

_____

Copyright © 2006. Lippincott Williams & Wilkins. *Study Guide to Accompany Essentials of Nursing Research,* by Denise F. Polit and Cheryl Tatano Beck.

■ The infants in which of the three treatment groups weighed the most, on average?

_____

_____

■ Which group was most homogeneous with respect to severity of illness (i.e., scores on the SNAP: PE)? Which group was most heterogeneous?

_____

_____

b. According to the text, were any of the group differences on baseline characteristics statistically significant? What does this mean?

_____

_____

c. Answer the following questions about the test of the main study hypotheses:

■ For the main study hypotheses, what were the independent and dependent variables?

_____

_____

■ What statistical test was used to test the main study hypotheses?

_____

_____

■ What was the between-subjects factor? What was the within-subjects factor? Which of these two factors was the principal test?

_____

_____

■ Were the main effects statistically significant? If so, at what probability level? What was the value of F for the between-groups factor? What was the probability level for the between-groups factor?

_____

_____

■ Was the interaction effect statistically significant? What is the probability that the interaction of time and groups was spurious?

_____

_____

Copyright © 2006. Lippincott Williams & Wilkins. _Study Guide to Accompany Essentials of Nursing Research_, by Denise F. Polit and Cheryl Tatano Beck.

■ Why did the researchers perform post hoc tests? What did the tests indicate?

_____

_____

■ What do the results of the main statistical tests mean?

_____

_____

d. Referring to Table 2, answer the following questions:

■ Which two descriptive statistics are presented in this table?

_____

_____

■ Does the table itself present any inferential statistics?

_____

_____

■ Which group had the highest PIPP score at 30 seconds?

_____

_____

■ Which group had the smallest amount of change in PIPP scores between 30 seconds and 60 seconds?

_____

_____

■ Variability in PIPP scores was lowest for which group, at which time?

_____

_____

e. Answer the following questions about the multiple regression analysis:

■ What was the dependent variable?

_____

_____

■ What were the independent variables?

_____

_____

Copyright © 2006. Lippincott Williams & Wilkins. _Study Guide to Accompany Essentials of Nursing Research,_ by Denise F. Polit and Cheryl Tatano Beck.

■ Which of the independent variables were found to be significant predictors of PIPP scores?

_____

_____

■ Was the value of R^2 indicated? If so, what was it?

_____

_____

QUESTIONS FOR DISCUSSION

a. Discuss the effectiveness of the presentation of information in the tables. What, if anything, could be done to make the tables more informative, clear, or efficient? Should there have been other tables?

_____

_____

b. Did the researchers use the appropriate statistical tests to analyze their data? If not, what tests should have been performed?

_____

_____

c. Did the researchers present a sufficient amount of information about their statistical tests? What additional information would have been helpful?

_____

_____

2. Read the results section of the report by Loeb ("Older Men's Health") in Appendix C. Then answer the following questions:

QUESTIONS OF FACT

a. Referring to Table 1, answer the following questions:

■ What is the correlation between the men's Healthiness of Lifestyle scores and Health-Promoting Behaviors (HPAOAM) scores?

_____

_____

Copyright © 2006. Lippincott Williams & Wilkins. *Study Guide to Accompany Essentials of Nursing Research*, by Denise F. Polit and Cheryl Tatano Beck.

■ What variables are negatively correlated with the variable "Total screenings"?

_____

_____

■ Scores on the HSDI (Health motivation) were significantly correlated with which other variables?

_____

_____

■ What is the strongest correlation in this matrix? What is the probability level associated with it?

_____

_____

■ What is the weakest correlation in this matrix? What is the probability associated with it?

_____

_____

■ What is the name of the test statistic presented in this table?

_____

_____

■ Are any of the variables in this table nominal-level measures?

_____

_____

■ According to this table, are older men who attended more health-promoting programs significantly more likely than other men to participate in appropriate health screenings?

_____

_____

b. Referring to Table 2 and the accompanying text, answer the following questions:

■ What was the dependent variable in the multiple regression analysis?

_____

_____

Copyright © 2006. Lippincott Williams & Wilkins. *Study Guide to Accompany Essentials of Nursing Research*, by Denise F. Polit and Cheryl Tatano Beck.

■ Which predictor variable was most strongly correlated with the dependent variable?

_____

_____

■ What was the value of R^2 after the first variable entered the regression equation?

_____

_____

■ How many predictor variables in total were used in the final regression equation, as shown in the table?

_____

_____

■ Were there other variables that Loeb tried to include in the regression analysis? Why were these variables not used?

_____

_____

■ What was the final value of R^2?

_____

_____

c. Referring to Table 3 and the accompanying text, answer the following questions:

■ What is the independent variable in the analyses presented in this table?

_____

_____

■ What statistical test was used in the analyses presented in this table?

_____

_____

■ Which group had higher average scores on the HSDI? Was the group difference statistically significant? What does this mean?

_____

_____

Copyright © 2006. Lippincott Williams & Wilkins. _Study Guide to Accompany Essentials of Nursing Research_, by Denise F. Polit and Cheryl Tatano Beck.

■ For which dependent variables were the groups significantly different?

_____

_____

d. The title of Table 4 is incorrect. What should it be?

_____

_____

QUESTIONS FOR DISCUSSION

a. Discuss the effectiveness of the presentation of information in the tables. What, if anything, could be done to make the tables more informative, clear, or efficient? Should there have been other tables?

_____

_____

b. Did Loeb use the appropriate statistical tests to analyze her data? If not, what tests should have been performed?

_____

_____

c. Did Loeb present a sufficient amount of information about her statistical tests? What additional information would have been helpful?

_____

_____

Copyright © 2006. Lippincott Williams & Wilkins. *Study Guide to Accompany Essentials of Nursing Research*, by Denise F. Polit and Cheryl Tatano Beck.

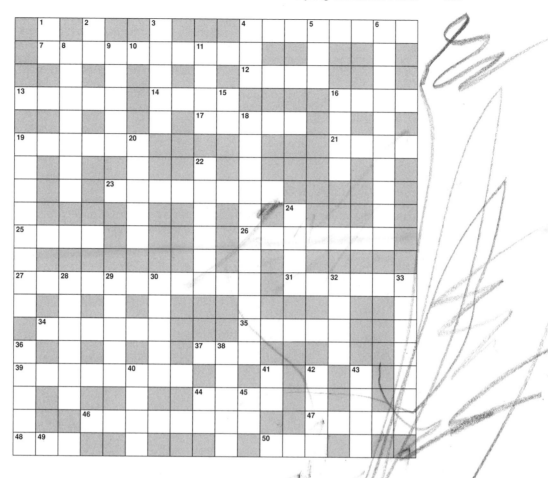

ACROSS

4. The most common index of variability is the _____ deviation.

7. ANCOVA is an acronym for analysis of _____.

12. The sum of scores divided by sample size yields a(n) _____.

13. In a *t*-test, the _____ variable is a nominal-level variable (abbr.).

14. In a crosstabulation, the intersection of a row and a column is a(n) _____.

16. A descriptive index (e.g., an average) for a population (abbr.)

17. The _____ of significance establishes the risk of making a type I error.

19. LISREL is an acronym for _____ structural relation analysis.

21. In using inferential statistics, researchers must compute a(n) _____ statistic.

23. MANOVA is an acronym for multivariate _____ of variance.

Copyright © 2006. Lippincott Williams & Wilkins. *Study Guide to Accompany Essentials of Nursing Research,* by Denise F. Polit and Cheryl Tatano Beck.

25. Distributions with a tail pointing to the left have a negative _____.

26. In ANOVA, _____ -group variability is contrasted with within-group variability.

27. The broad class of statistics used to draw conclusions about a population

31. To determine significance, a computed test statistic is compared to a _____ value for a theoretical distribution.

34. The multivariate procedure used to reduce a large set of variables to a smaller set is _____ analysis.

35. The statistical test used to compare two group means

37. Means from a factorial experiment could be analyzed using a two-_____ ANOVA.

39. Distributions with a single high point

44. After an ANOVA, researchers perform _____ hoc tests.

46. The statistic $r = .85$ indicates a strong, _____ relationship between two variables.

47. A bimodal distribution has two _____.

48. Another terms for a negative relationship is a(n) _____ relationship (abbr.).

50. The mean is the _____ of all values, divided by number of subjects.

DOWN

1. The index summarizing the direction and strength of a relationship (acronym)

2. The variable being predicted in a multiple regression (acronym)

3. A multivariate procedure for predicting group membership (abbr.)

4. The standard deviation in a sampling distribution of means (acronym)

5. Inferential statistics without rigorous assumptions about distributional properties are _____ parametric.

6. Multiple _____ analysis could be used to predict blood pressure based on multiple predictors.

8. The level of measurement involving rank ordering but not equal distances

9. The risk of a type I error

10. The statistic representing a Pearson product-moment correlation coefficient

11. A type I error involves rejection of a true _____ hypothesis.

15. In the expression $p \leq .05$, the symbol $\leq$ is sometimes abbreviated ___ ___.

16. A(n) _____ analysis is an approach to causal modeling.

Copyright © 2006. Lippincott Williams & Wilkins. *Study Guide to Accompany Essentials of Nursing Research*, by Denise F. Polit and Cheryl Tatano Beck.

18. The range and SD are measures of _____.

19. A _____ regression uses an alternative estimation procedure to predict a nominal-level dependent variable from multiple predictors.

20. The highest score value minus the lowest score value

22. The error committed when a false null hypothesis is accepted

24. A descriptive index (e.g., an average) for a sample (abbr.)

28. The statistic computed in analysis of variance

29. The highest level of measurement

30. A bell-shaped curve is a popular name for a _____ l distribution.

32. The risk of making a type II error

33. The number of observations free to vary about a parameter are the _____ of freedom.

36. A distribution with two or more peaks is _____ modal.

38. The test used to compare three or more group means (acronym)

40. The class of statistics used to summarize data, not to estimate population parameters (abbr.)

41. In the expression $p > .05$, the symbol $>$ is sometimes abbreviated _____.

42. A distribution without a skew is a _____ distribution (abbr.).

43. The ratio of two probabilities—the likelihood of occurrence versus nonoccurrence, which can be expressed as a ratio

44. A constant, used to compute the area of a circle

45. Acronym for standard error

46. The probability that obtained results are due to chance is expressed by a(n) _____ value.

49. Symbol designating total sample size

Copyright © 2006. Lippincott Williams & Wilkins. *Study Guide to Accompany Essentials of Nursing Research*, by Denise F. Polit and Cheryl Tatano Beck.

CHAPTER 16

Analyzing Qualitative Data

■ A. Matching Exercises

1. *Match each descriptive statement from Set B with one or more types of qualitative analysis from Set A. Indicate the letter(s) corresponding to your response next to each item in Set B.*

SET A

a. Grounded theory analysis
b. Phenomenological/hermeneutic analysis
c. Ethnographic analysis
d. None of the above

SET B   **RESPONSES**

1. Involves the development of coding categories   _____

2. Begins with "open coding"   _____

3. The method of analysis developed by Colaizzi   _____

4. Data can be organized using computer software   _____

5. The method of analysis developed by Glaser and Strauss   _____

6. May involve the development of a taxonomy   _____

7. One analytic approach involves identifying paradigm cases.   _____

8. Often uses a style most likely to be described as "template analysis style"   _____

9. Often uses a style most likely to be described as "editing analysis style"   _____

10. Requires the use of quasi-statistics   _____

Copyright © 2006. Lippincott Williams & Wilkins. *Study Guide to Accompany Essentials of Nursing Research*, by Denise F. Polit and Cheryl Tatano Beck.

■ B. Completion Exercises

Write the words or phrases that correctly complete the sentences below.

1. Data collection and data analysis typically occur _____

   _____ in qualitative studies, not as separate phases.

2. The four processes that play a role in qualitative analysis are _____,

   _____, _____, and _____.

3. The main task in organizing qualitative data involves the development of a method of

   _____ and _____ the data.

4. A(n) _____

   is a physical file that is organized to contain all material relating to a topic area.

5. Traditional methods of organizing qualitative data are being replaced by _____

   _____.

6. The analysis of qualitative data generally begins with a search for _____

   _____.

7. The use of _____ involves an accounting of

   the frequency with which certain themes and relationships are supported by the data.

8. The four levels of analysis in Spradley's ethnographic method are _____

   _____ analysis, _____ analysis, _____

   analysis, and _____ analysis.

9. Colaizzi, Giorgi, and Van Kaam's methods of analysis are used to analyze data from a

   study in the _____ tradition.

10. One of Van Manen's approaches to data analysis is referred to as the _____

    _____ approach, which involves an analysis of every sentence of data.

11. In the approach espoused by Diekelmann and colleagues, the highest level of

    hermeneutic analysis involves the discovery of a(n) _____.

12. In Benner's interpretive approach, _____ are used early in the

    analytic process as a means of gaining understanding about the central phenomenon.

13. In grounded theory, the process of breaking down the data, examining them, and

    comparing them to other segments is referred to as _____

    _____.

Copyright © 2006. Lippincott Williams & Wilkins. *Study Guide to Accompany Essentials of Nursing Research*, by Denise F. Polit and Cheryl Tatano Beck.

14. In a grounded theory study, the initial phase of coding is referred to as _____
_____.

15. In grounded theory studies, coding of information relating only to the core variable
is referred to as _____ coding.

16. A particular type of core variable in a grounded theory study is the _____
_____ or BSP.

■ C. Study Questions

1. Complete the crossword puzzle at the end of the chapter, which uses terms and concepts presented in Chapter 16. (Puzzles may be removed for easier viewing.)

2. What is wrong with the following statements?

   a. Hall conducted a grounded theory study about coping with a miscarriage in which
   she was able to identify four major themes.

   _____

   _____

   b. Lowe's ethnographic analysis of Haitian clinics involved gleaning related thematic
   material from French poetry.

   _____

   _____

   c. Allen's phenomenological study of the lived experience of Parkinson's disease
   focused on the domain of fatigue.

   _____

   _____

   d. Dodd's grounded theory study of widowhood yielded a taxonomy of coping strategies.

   _____

   _____

   e. In her ethnographic study of the culture of a nursing home, MacLean used a rural
   nursing home as a paradigm case.

   _____

   _____

3. Which of the following would lend themselves to a visual display of the findings (for
example, like Figure 1 in Bent's study, "Empowerment Process," Appendix D)? Justify
your response.

Copyright © 2006. Lippincott Williams & Wilkins. *Study Guide to Accompany Essentials
of Nursing Research*, by Denise F. Polit and Cheryl Tatano Beck.

■ A taxonomy
■ A BSP
■ A paradigm case
■ A hermeneutic circle

_____

_____

_____

_____

_____

4. In the study in Appendix B ("Homeless Youth"), Rew presented a list of study participants and some of their demographic and identifying characteristics (Table 1). Instead of using a table, Rew could have described the sample in paragraph form. Try writing a short paragraph describing a segment of the sample (i.e., the males or the females, the minorities or the whites, etc.).

■ D. Application Exercises

1. Read the "data analysis" and results sections of the report by Rew ("Homeless Youth") in Appendix B. Then answer the following questions:

QUESTIONS OF FACT

a. How many pages of transcribed interview data did the study yield? How many pages of field notes were there?

_____

_____

b. Was constant comparison used in analyzing the data?

_____

_____

c. Did Rew create conceptual files?

_____

_____

d. Was a computer used to analyze the data? If yes, what software was used?

_____

_____

Copyright © 2006. Lippincott Williams & Wilkins. _Study Guide to Accompany Essentials of Nursing Research,_ by Denise F. Polit and Cheryl Tatano Beck.

e. Did Rew calculate any quasi-statistics?

_____

_____

f. Which grounded theory analytic approach was adopted in this study?

_____

_____

g. Did Rew prepare any analytic memos?

_____

_____

h. Did Rew describe the open coding process? If so, what did she say?

_____

_____

i. Did Rew describe axial coding? If so, what did she say?

_____

_____

j. How many categories initially emerged in Rew's analysis?

_____

_____

k. How many major categories were ultimately developed and refined? What were they?

_____

_____

l. What was the BSP? What does the BSP entail?

_____

_____

QUESTIONS FOR DISCUSSION

a. Discuss the thoroughness of Rew's description of her data analysis efforts. Did the report present adequate information about the coding of the data and the steps taken to analyze the data?

_____

_____

Copyright © 2006. Lippincott Williams & Wilkins. *Study Guide to Accompany Essentials of Nursing Research,* by Denise F. Polit and Cheryl Tatano Beck.

b. Was there any evidence of "method slurring"—that is, did Rew consistently apply analytic procedures that are appropriate for a grounded theory approach?

_____

_____

c. Discuss the effectiveness of Rew's presentation of results. Does the analysis seem sensible, thoughtful, and thorough? Was sufficient evidence provided to support the findings? Were data presented in a manner that allows you to be confident about Rew's conclusions?

_____

_____

d. Did the model in Figure 1 effectively display the grounded theory? Did it adequately communicate the core variable?

_____

_____

2. Read the "data analysis" and "findings" sections of the report by Bent ("Empowerment Process") in Appendix D. Then answer the following questions:

QUESTIONS OF FACT

a. How many pages of transcribed interview data did the study yield? How many pages of field notes did the study yield?

_____

_____

b. Was constant comparison used in analyzing the data?

_____

_____

c. Did Bent create conceptual files?

_____

_____

d. Was a computer used to analyze the data? If yes, what software was used?

_____

_____

Copyright © 2006. Lippincott Williams & Wilkins. *Study Guide to Accompany Essentials of Nursing Research*, by Denise F. Polit and Cheryl Tatano Beck.

e. Did Bent calculate any quasi-statistics?

_____

_____

f. Was Spradley's method of ethnographic analysis used in this study?

_____

_____

g. Did Bent describe the coding process? If so, what did she say?

_____

_____

h. Did Bent identify any domains? If so, how many and what were they?

_____

_____

i. Did Bent create a taxonomy or undertake a taxonomic analysis? If yes, what did the taxonomy encompass?

_____

_____

j. Did Bent undertake a theme analysis? If yes, what were the cultural themes?

_____

_____

QUESTIONS FOR DISCUSSION

a. Discuss the thoroughness of Bent's description of her data analysis efforts. Did the report present adequate information about the coding of the data and the steps taken to analyze the data?

_____

_____

b. Was there any evidence of "method slurring"—that is, did Bent consistently apply analytic procedures that are appropriate for an ethnography?

_____

_____

Copyright © 2006. Lippincott Williams & Wilkins. *Study Guide to Accompany Essentials of Nursing Research*, by Denise F. Polit and Cheryl Tatano Beck.

c. Discuss the effectiveness of Bent's presentation of results. Does the analysis seem sensible, thoughtful, and thorough? Was sufficient evidence provided to support the findings? Were data presented in a manner that allows you to be confident about Bent's conclusions?

_____

_____

d. Did the model in Figure 1 effectively display the ethnographic findings? Did the model emerge from Bent's data?

_____

_____

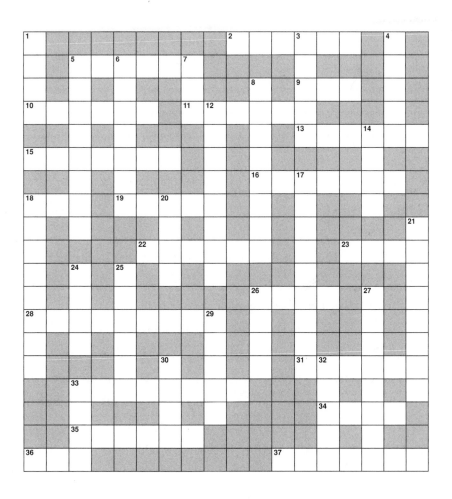

ACROSS

2. Colaizzi's method involves the use of _____ checks.

5. Phenomenological analysis involves the identification of essential _____.

9. In Glaser & Strauss's method, there are theoretical codes and _____ codes (abbr.).

10. In ethnographies, a broad unit of cultural knowledge

11. In vivo codes, first coding step in grounded theory

13. The hermeneutic _____ involves movement between the parts and whole of a text being analyzed.

15. _____ i was a prominent analyst and writer in the Duquesne school of phenomenology.

16. The discovery of a constitutive _____ forms the highest level of analysis in Diekelmann's approach.

18. In grounded theory, the process of identifying characteristics of one piece of data and comparing them with those of another to determine similarity

19. The phenomenologist _____ i did not espouse validating themes with peers or study participants.

22. The hermeneutic approach of _____ includes an analysis of exemplars.

23. Transcribed interviews are usually the main form of _____ in phenomenological analysis.

26. Timelines and _____ charts are devices used to highlight time sequences in qualitative analysis. ·

28. The most interpretive and subjective qualitative analysis styles

31. After a categorization system is developed, the main task involves _____ the data.

33. A Dutch phenomenologist who encouraged the use of artistic sources

34. Sometimes the analysis of qualitative _____ is described as content analysis.

35. Before analysis can begin, qualitative researchers have to develop a categorization _____.

36. All of a phenomenologist's transcribed interviews would comprise a qualitative data _____.

37. One of the two major schools of phenomenology

Copyright © 2006. Lippincott Williams & Wilkins. *Study Guide to Accompany Essentials of Nursing Research*, by Denise F. Polit and Cheryl Tatano Beck.

DOWN

1. A recurring _____ in a set of interviews can be the basis for an emerging theme.

3. One type of core variable in grounded theory is a _____ social process that evolves over time.

4. A type of coding in Strauss and Corbin's approach wherein the analyst links subcategories

5. A guide for sorting narrative data, often drafted before analysis begins

6. Grounded theorists and phenomenologists typically use this broad type of qualitative analysis style.

7. The type of coding of data relating to the core variable in grounded theory (abbr.)

8. Sometimes used to enrich an analytic strategy, especially by interpretive phenomenologists

12. Themes and conceptualizations are viewed as _____ from the data in qualitative analysis.

14. In grounded theory, the _____ category is a central pattern that is relevant to participants.

17. The second level of analysis in Spradley's ethnographic method

18. Glaser proposed 18 _____ of theoretical codes to help grounded theorists conceptualize relationships.

20. The first stage of constant comparison involves _____ coding.

21. Strong examples of ways of being in the world are _____ cases.

24. Grounded theorists document an idea in an analytic _____.

25. The nurse researcher who developed an alternative approach to grounded theory analysis

26. In manual organization of qualitative data, excerpts are cut up and inserted into a conceptual _____.

27. In Van Manen's _____ approach, the analyst sees the text as a whole and tries to capture its meaning.

Copyright © 2006. Lippincott Williams & Wilkins. *Study Guide to Accompany Essentials of Nursing Research*, by Denise F. Polit and Cheryl Tatano Beck.

29. The field _____ of an ethnographer are an important source of data for analysis.

30. Van _____ was a phenomenologist from the Duquesne school.

32. The point of developing a system of categorization is to impose _____ on the narrative information.

33. The amount of data collected in a typical qualitative study typically is _____.

Copyright © 2006. Lippincott Williams & Wilkins. *Study Guide to Accompany Essentials of Nursing Research*, by Denise F. Polit and Cheryl Tatano Beck.

PART 6

Critical Appraisal and Utilization of Nursing Research

CHAPTER 17

Critiquing Research Reports

■ A. Matching Exercises

1. *Match each of the questions in Set B with the research decision for quantitative studies being evaluated, as listed in Set A. Indicate the letter corresponding to your response next to each of the statements in Set B.*

SET A

a. Research design decisions

b. The population and sampling plan

c. Data collection procedures

d. Analytic decisions

SET B   **RESPONSES**

1. Was there a sufficient number of subjects?   _____

2. Was there evidence of adequate reliability and validity?   _____

3. Would a more limited specification have controlled some
   extraneous variables not covered by the research design?   _____

4. Would multivariate procedures have been more appropriate?   _____

5. Should a power analysis have been used to determine size?   _____

6. Were threats to internal validity adequately controlled?   _____

7. Were the statistical tests appropriate, given the level of
   measurement of the variables?   _____

8. Were response set biases minimized?   _____

9. Was the comparison group equivalent to the experimental group?   _____

10. Should the data have been collected prospectively?   _____

2. *Match each of the questions in Set B with the research decision for qualitative studies being evaluated, as listed in Set A. Indicate the letter corresponding to your response next to each of the statements in Set B.*

Copyright © 2006. Lippincott Williams & Wilkins. *Study Guide to Accompany Essentials of Nursing Research*, by Denise F. Polit and Cheryl Tatano Beck.

SET A

a. The setting

b. Data sources and data quality

c. Sampling plan

d. Data analysis

SET B   **RESPONSES**

1. Were triangulation procedures used as a method of validation?   _____

2. Was there a sufficient number of study participants to achieve
   saturation?   _____

3. Were constant comparison procedures appropriately used to
   refine relevant categories?   _____

4. Were the interviews of sufficient depth?   _____

5. Were participants asked to comment on the emerging themes?   _____

6. Did the study take place in an information-rich location?   _____

7. Were the study participants the best possible informants?   _____

8. Do the themes seem parsimonious, logical, and nonsuperficial?   _____

■ B. Completion Exercises

Write the words or phrases that correctly complete the sentences below.

1. The first step in the interpretation of research findings involves an analysis of the

   _____ of the results,

   based on various types of evidence.

2. Interpretation of quantitative results is easiest when the results are consistent with

   the researcher's _____.

3. An important research precept is that correlation does not prove _____

   _____.

4. Researchers should avoid the temptation of going beyond _____

   _____.

5. Statistical significance does not necessarily mean that research results are _____

   _____.

Copyright © 2006. Lippincott Williams & Wilkins. *Study Guide to Accompany Essentials
of Nursing Research,* by Denise F. Polit and Cheryl Tatano Beck.

6. The research process involves numerous methodologic _____

_____, each of which could affect

the quality of the study.

7. A good critique should identify both _____ and

_____ in a study.

8. An evaluation of the relevance of a study to some aspect of the nursing profession

involves critiquing the _____

_____ dimension of a research study.

9. An evaluation of the researcher's study design involves critiquing the _____

_____ dimension of a research study.

10. An evaluation of the way in which human subjects were treated involves critiquing the

_____

dimension of a research study.

11. An evaluation of the sense the researcher tried to make of the results involves critiquing

the _____ dimension of

the research study.

12. An evaluation of the conciseness and organization of the research report involves

critiquing the _____

_____ dimension of the research study.

■ C. Study Questions

1. Complete the crossword puzzle at the end of the chapter, which uses terms and concepts presented in Chapter 17. (Puzzles may be removed for easier viewing.)

2. Read the following qualitative research report and identify the study's major strengths and limitations:

   Salazar, M. K., Napolitano, M., Scherer, J. A., & McCauley, L. A. (2004). Hispanic adolescent farmworkers' perceptions associated with pesticide exposure. *Western Journal of Nursing Research, 26,* 146–166.

   Now, read the two commentaries of the study that immediately follow the report (pages 167–172). Do any of your comments overlap with those of the commentators? Do you agree or disagree with either or both sets of comments?

Copyright © 2006. Lippincott Williams & Wilkins. *Study Guide to Accompany Essentials of Nursing Research,* by Denise F. Polit and Cheryl Tatano Beck.

3. Read and critique one or more of the articles below (or other articles in the nursing research literature), and apply the questions in Box 17-4 of the textbook to the article. Prepare two to three pages of "bullet points" that indicate the major strengths and weaknesses of the study.

Quantitative Studies

Bliss, D. Z., Fischer, L. R., Savik, K., Avery, M., & Mark, P. (2004). Severity of fecal incontinence in community-living elderly in a health maintenance organization. *Research in Nursing & Health, 27*, 162–173.

Macnee, C. L., & McCabe, S. (2004). The transtheoretical model of behavior change and smokers in southern Appalachia. *Nursing Research, 53*, 243–250.

Miller, K. H., & Grindel, C. G. (2004). Comparison of symptoms of younger and older patients undergoing coronary artery bypass surgery. *Clinical Nursing Research, 13*, 179–193.

Qualitative Studies

Finfgeld-Connett, D. (2005). Telephone support or nursing presence? Analysis of a nursing intervention. *Qualitative Health Research, 15*, 19–29.

Montbriand, M. J. (2004). Seniors' life histories and perceptions of illness. *Western Journal of Nursing Research, 26*, 242–260.

O'Reilly, M. M. (2004). Achieving a new balance: Women's transition to second-time parenthood. *Journal of Obstetric, Gynecologic, & Neonatal Nursing, 33*, 455–462.

■ D. Application Exercises

1. Read the discussion section by Gibbins and colleagues ("Procedural Pain") in Appendix A. Then answer the following questions:

QUESTIONS OF FACT

a. Did the researchers discuss all of their findings?

_____

_____

b. Did the researchers link the findings of their study to findings from earlier studies? If yes, were the findings of this study consistent with findings from other studies?

_____

_____

Copyright © 2006. Lippincott Williams & Wilkins. *Study Guide to Accompany Essentials of Nursing Research*, by Denise F. Polit and Cheryl Tatano Beck.

c. Did the researchers discuss any limitations of the study?

_____

_____

d. Did the researchers make any distinction between clinical and statistical significance?

_____

_____

e. Did the researchers discuss the implications of the study for practice?

_____

_____

f. Did the researchers make any recommendations for further research?

_____

_____

QUESTIONS FOR DISCUSSION

a. Were there study limitations that the researchers did not discuss, but should have?

_____

_____

b. Are the researchers' interpretations consistent with the results? Do the interpretations suggest any biases? Do the researchers "go beyond their data"?

_____

_____

2. Below is a fictitious research report and a critique of various aspects of it. This example is designed to highlight features about the form and content of both a written report and a written evaluation of the study's worth. To economize on space, the report is brief, but it incorporates essential elements for a meaningful appraisal.

   Read the report and critique, and then determine whether you agree with the critique. Can you add other comments relevant to a critical appraisal of the study?

Copyright © 2006. Lippincott Williams & Wilkins. _Study Guide to Accompany Essentials of Nursing Research_, by Denise F. Polit and Cheryl Tatano Beck.

The Role of Health Care Providers in Teenage Pregnancy

by Phyllis Clinton

Background. Of the 20 million teenagers living in the United States, about one in four is sexually active by age 14; more than half have had sexual intercourse by age 17 (Kelman & Saner, 1998).[1] Despite increased availability of contraceptives, the number of teenage pregnancies has remained fairly stable over the past 2 decades. About 1 million girls under age 20 become pregnant each year and, of these, about 500,000 become teenaged mothers (U. S. Bureau of the Census, 1998).

Public concern regarding teenage pregnancy stems not only from the high rates, but also from the extensive research that has documented the adverse consequences of early parenthood in the health arena. Pregnant teenagers have been found to receive less prenatal care (Tremain, 2000), to be more likely to develop toxemia (Schendley, 1991; Waters, 1999), to be more likely to experience prolonged labor (Curran, 1989), to be more likely to have low-birth-weight babies (Tremain, 2000; Beach, 1995), and to be at increased risk of having babies with low Apgar scores (Beach, 1995) than older mothers. The long-term consequences to the teenaged mothers themselves are also extremely bleak: Teenaged mothers get less schooling, are more likely to be on public assistance, tend to earn lower wages, and are more likely to get divorced if they marry than their peers who postpone parenthood (Jamail, 1999; North, 1992; Smithfield, 1991).

The 1 million teenagers who become pregnant each year are caught up in a tough emotional decision—to carry the pregnancy to term and keep the baby, to have an abortion, or to deliver the baby and surrender it for adoption. Despite the widely reported adverse consequences of young parenthood cited above, most young women today are opting for delivery and child-rearing, often out of wedlock (Jaffrey, 1994; Henderson, 2001). Relatively few young mothers in recent years have been relinquishing their babies for adoption, forcing many couples with fertility problems to seek adoption options overseas (Smith, 1998).

The purpose of this study was to test the effect of a special intervention based in an outpatient clinic of a Chicago hospital on improving the health outcomes of a group of pregnant teenagers. Specifically, it was hypothesized that pregnant teenagers who were in the special program would receive more prenatal care, be less likely to develop toxemia, be less likely to have a low-birth-weight baby, spend fewer hours in labor, have babies with higher Apgar scores, and be more likely to use a contraceptive at 6 months postpartum than pregnant teenagers not enrolled in the program.

The theoretical model on which this research was based is an ecologic model of personal behavior (Brandenburg, 1984). A schematic diagram of the ecologic model is presented in Figure 17-A. In this framework, the actions of the person are the focus of attention, but those actions are believed to be a function not only of the person's own characteristics, attitudes,

---

[1]All references in this example are fictitious, although most of the information in this fictitious literature review is based on real studies.

Copyright © 2006. Lippincott Williams & Wilkins. *Study Guide to Accompany Essentials of Nursing Research*, by Denise F. Polit and Cheryl Tatano Beck.

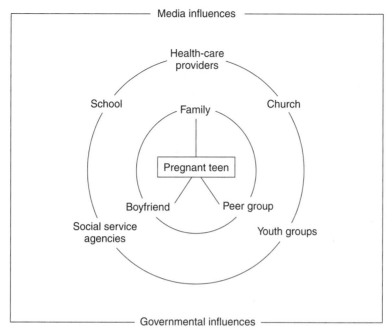

FIGURE 17-A Model of ecologic contexts

and abilities, but also of other influences in their environment. Environmental influences can be differentiated according to their proximal relationship with the target person. Health care workers and institutions are, according to the model, more distant influences than family, peers, and boyfriends. Yet it is assumed that these less immediate forces are real and can intervene to change the behaviors of the target person. Thus, it is hypothesized that pregnant teenagers can be influenced by increased exposure to a health care team providing a structured program of services designed to promote improved health outcomes.

Method. A special program of services for pregnant teenagers was implemented in the outpatient clinic of an inner-city public hospital in Chicago. The intervention involved 8 weeks of nutrition education and counseling, parenting education, instruction on prenatal health care, preparation for childbirth, and contraceptive counseling.

All teenagers with a confirmed pregnancy attending the clinic were asked if they wanted to participate in the special program. The goal was to enroll 150 pregnant teenagers during the program's first year of operation. A total of 276 teenagers attending the clinic were invited to participate; of these, 59 had an abortion or miscarriage and 108 declined to participate, yielding an experimental group sample of 109 girls.

To test the effectiveness of the special program, a comparison group of pregnant teenagers was needed. Another inner-city hospital agreed to cooperate in the study. Staff obtained information on the labor and delivery outcomes of the 120 teenagers who delivered at the comparison hospital, where no special teen-parent program was available. For both experimental group and comparison group subjects, a follow-up telephone interview was conducted 6 months postpartum to determine if the teenagers were using birth control.

Copyright © 2006. Lippincott Williams & Wilkins. *Study Guide to Accompany Essentials of Nursing Research*, by Denise F. Polit and Cheryl Tatano Beck.

The outcome variables in this study were the teenagers' labor and delivery and postpartum outcomes and their contraceptive behavior. Operational definitions of these variables were as follows:

Prenatal care: Number of visits made to a physician or nurse during the pregnancy, exclusive of the visit for the pregnancy test

Toxemia: Presence versus absence of preeclamptic toxemia as diagnosed by a physician

Labor time: Number of hours elapsed from the first contractions until delivery of the baby, to the nearest half hour

Low infant birth weight: Infant birth weights of less than 2500 grams versus those of 2500 grams or greater

Apgar score: Infant Apgar score (from 0 to 10) taken at 3 minutes after birth

Contraceptive use postpartum: Self-reported use of any form of birth control 6 months postpartum versus self-reported nonuse

The two groups were compared on these six outcome measures using t-tests and chi-squared tests.

Results. The teenagers in the sample were, on average, 17.6 years old at the time of delivery. The mean age was 17.0 in the experimental group and 18.1 in the comparison group ($p < .05$).

By definition, all the teenagers in the experimental group had received prenatal care. Two of the teenagers in the comparison group had no health care treatment before delivery. The distribution of visits for the two groups is presented in Figure 17-B. The experimental group had a higher mean number of prenatal visits than the comparison group, as shown in Table 17-A, but the difference was not statistically significant at the .05 level, using a t-test for independent groups.

In the sample as a whole, about 1 girl in 10 was diagnosed as having preeclamptic toxemia. The difference between the two groups was in the hypothesized direction, with 1.6% more of the comparison group teenagers developing this complication, but the difference was not significant using a χ^2 test.

The hours spent in labor ranged from 3.5 to 29.0 in the experimental group and from 4.5 to 33.5 in the comparison group. On average, teenagers in the experimental group spent 14.3 hours in labor, compared with 15.2 for the comparison group teenagers. The difference was not statistically significant.

With regard to low-birth-weight babies, a total of 43 girls out of 229 in the sample gave birth to babies who weighed under 2500 grams (5.5 pounds).[2] More of the comparison group teenagers (20.9%) than experimental group teenagers (16.5%) had low-birth-weight babies, but, once again, the group difference was not significant.

The 3-minute Apgar score in the two groups was quite similar—7.3 for the experimental group and 6.7 for the comparison group. This difference was nonsignificant.

---

[2]All mothers gave birth to live infants; however, there were two neonatal deaths within 24 hours of birth in the comparison group.

Copyright © 2006. Lippincott Williams & Wilkins. *Study Guide to Accompany Essentials of Nursing Research*, by Denise F. Polit and Cheryl Tatano Beck.

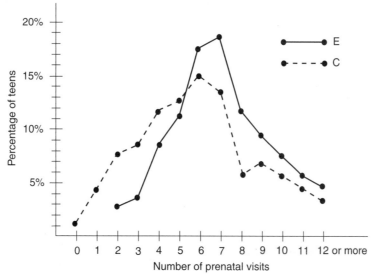

FIGURE 17-B Frequency distribution of prenatal visits, by experimental versus comparison group. (*E*, experimental group; *C*, comparison group)

TABLE 17-A Summary of Experimental and Comparison Group Differences

Outcome Variable	Group Experimental ($n = 109$)	Comparison ($n = 120$)	Difference	Test Statistic
Mean number of prenatal visits	7.1	5.9	1.2	$t = 1.83$, $df = 227$, NS
Percentage with toxemia	10.1%	11.7%	−1.6%	$\chi^2 = 0.15$, $df = 1$, NS
Mean hours spent in labor	14.3	15.2	−.09	$t = 1.01$, $df = 227$, NS
Percentage with low-birth-weight baby	16.5%	20.9%	−4.4%	$\chi^2 = 0.71$, $df = 1$, NS
Mean Apgar score	7.3	6.7	.6	$t = 0.98$, $df = 227$, NS
Percentage adopting contraception post-partum	81.7%	62.5%	19.2%	$\chi^2 = 10.22$, $df = 1$, $p < .01$

Copyright © 2006. Lippincott Williams & Wilkins. *Study Guide to Accompany Essentials of Nursing Research*, by Denise F. Polit and Cheryl Tatano Beck.

Finally, the teenagers were compared with respect to their use of birth control 6 months after delivering their babies. For this variable, teenagers were coded as users of contraception if they were either using some method of birth control at the time of the follow-up interview or if they were nonusers but were sexually inactive (*i.e.*, were using abstinence to prevent a repeat pregnancy). The results of the χ^2 test revealed that a significantly higher percentage of experimental group teenagers (81.7%) than comparison group teenagers (62.5%) reported using birth control after delivery. This difference was significant beyond the .01 level.

Discussion. The results of this evaluation were disappointing, but not discouraging. There was only one outcome for which a significant difference was observed. The experimental program significantly increased the percentage of teenagers who used birth control after delivering their babies. Thus, one highly important result of participating in the program is that an early repeat pregnancy will be postponed. There is abundant research that has shown that repeat pregnancy among teenagers is especially damaging to their educational and occupational attainment and leads to particularly adverse labor and delivery outcomes in the higher-order births (Klugman, 1985; Jackson, 1997).

The experimental group had more prenatal care, but not significantly more. Perhaps part of the difficulty is that the program can only begin to deliver services once pregnancy has been diagnosed. If a teenager does not come in for a pregnancy test until her fourth or fifth month, this obviously puts an upper limit on the number of visits she will have; it also gives less time for her to eat properly, avoid smoking and drinking, and take other steps to enhance her health during pregnancy. Thus, one implication of this finding is that the program needs to do more to encourage early pregnancy screening. Perhaps a joint effort between the clinic personnel and school nurses in neighboring middle schools and high schools could be launched to publicize the need for a timely pregnancy test and to inform teenagers where such a test could be obtained. The two groups performed similarly with respect to the various labor and delivery outcomes chosen to evaluate the effectiveness of the new program. The issue of timeliness is again relevant here. The program may have been delivering services too late in the pregnancy for the instruction to have made much of an impact on the health of the mother and her child. This interpretation is supported, in part, by the fact that the one variable for which timeliness was *not* an issue (postpartum contraception) was, indeed, positively affected by program participation. Another possible implication is that the program itself should be made more powerful, for example, by lengthening or adding to instructional sessions.

Given that the experimental and comparison group differences were all in the hypothesized direction, it is also tempting to criticize the study's sample size. A larger sample (which was originally planned) might have yielded some significant differences.

In summary, the experimental intervention is not without promise. A particularly exciting finding is that participation in the program resulted in better contraceptive use, which will presumably lower the incidence of repeat pregnancy. It would be interesting to follow these teenagers 2 years after delivery to see if the groups differ in the rates of repeat pregnancy. It appears that more needs to be done to get these teenagers into the program early in their pregnancies. Perhaps then the true effectiveness of the program would be demonstrated.

Copyright © 2006. Lippincott Williams & Wilkins. *Study Guide to Accompany Essentials of Nursing Research*, by Denise F. Polit and Cheryl Tatano Beck.

Critique of the Research Report

In the following discussion, we present some comments on various aspects of this research report. You are urged to read the report and formulate your own opinion about its strengths and weaknesses before reading this critique. An evaluation of a study is necessarily partly subjective. Therefore, you might disagree with some of the points made below, and you might have additional criticisms and comments. We believe, however, that most of the serious methodologic flaws of the study are highlighted in our critique.

Title. The title for the study is misleading. The research does *not* investigate the role of health care professionals in serving the needs of pregnant teenagers. A more appropriate title would be "Health-Related Outcomes of an Intervention for Pregnant Teenagers."

Background. The background section of this report consists of three distinct elements that can be analyzed separately: a literature review, statement of the problem, and a theoretical framework.

The literature review is relatively clearly written and well-organized. It serves the important function of establishing a need for the experimental program by documenting the prevalence of teenage pregnancy and some of its adverse consequences. However, the literature review could be improved. First, an inspection of the citations suggests that the author is not as up-to-date on research relating to teenage pregnancy as she might have been. Most of the references are from the 1990s, meaning that this literature review is about a decade old. Second, there is material in the literature review section that is not relevant and should be removed. For example, the paragraph on the options with which a pregnant teenager is faced (paragraph 3) is not germane to the research problem. A third and more critical flaw is what the review does *not* cover. Given the research problem, there are probably four main points that should be addressed in the review:

1. How widespread is teenage pregnancy and parenthood?
2. What are the social and health consequences of early child-bearing?
3. What has been done (especially by nurses) to address the problems associated with teenage parenthood?
4. How successful have other interventions been?

The review adequately handles the first question: The need for concern is established. The second question is covered in the review, but perhaps more depth and more recent research is needed here. The new study is based on an assumption of negative health outcomes in teenaged mothers. The author has strung together a series of references without giving the reader any clues about the reliability of the information. Clinton would have made her point more convincingly if she had added a sentence such as, "For example, in a carefully executed prospective study involving nearly 8000 pregnant women, Beach (1995) found that young maternal age was significantly associated with higher rates of prematurity and other negative neonatal outcomes." The third and fourth points that should have been covered are totally absent from the review. Surely the author's experi-

Copyright © 2006. Lippincott Williams & Wilkins. *Study Guide to Accompany Essentials of Nursing Research,* by Denise F. Polit and Cheryl Tatano Beck.

mental program does not represent the first attempt to address the needs of pregnant teenagers. How is Clinton's intervention different from or better than other interventions? What reason does she have to believe that such an intervention might be successful? Clinton has provided a rationale for addressing the problem but no rationale for the manner in which she has addressed it. If, in fact, there is little information about other interventions and their effectiveness in improving health outcomes, then the review should say so.

The problem statement and hypothesis were stated succinctly and clearly. The hypothesis is complex (there are multiple dependent variables) and directional (it predicts better outcomes among teenagers participating in the special program).

The third component of the background section of the report is the theoretical framework. In our opinion, the theoretical framework chosen does little to enhance the research. The hypothesis is not generated on the basis of the model, nor does the intervention itself grow out of the model. One gets the feeling that the model was slapped on as an afterthought to try to make the study seem more sophisticated or theoretical. Actually, if more thought had been given to this conceptual framework, it might have proved useful. According to this model, the most immediate and direct influences on a pregnant teenager are her family, friends, and sexual partner. One programmatic implication of this is that the intervention should involve one or more of these influences. For example, a workshop for the teenagers' parents could have been developed to reinforce the teenagers' need for adequate nutrition and prenatal care. A research hypothesis that could have been tested in the context of the model is that teenagers who are missing one of the direct influences would be especially susceptible to the influence of less proximal health care providers (i.e., the program). For example, it might be hypothesized that pregnant teenagers who do not live with both parents have to depend on alternative sources of social support (such as health care personnel) during the pregnancy. Thus, it is not that the theoretical context selected is far-fetched, but rather that it was not convincingly linked to the actual research problem. Perhaps an alternative theoretical context would have been better. Or perhaps the researcher simply should have been honest and admitted that her research was practical, not theoretical.

Method. The design used to test the research hypothesis was a widely used preexperimental design. Two groups, whose equivalence is assumed but not established, were compared on several outcome measures. The design is one that has serious problems because the preintervention comparability of the groups is unknown.

The most serious threat to the internal validity of the study is selection bias. Selection bias can work both ways—either to mask true treatment effects or to create the illusion of a program effect when none exists. This is because selection bias can be either positive (i.e., the experimental group can be initially advantaged in relation to the comparison group) or negative (i.e., the experimental group can have pretreatment disadvantages). In the present study, it is possible that the two hospitals served clients of different economic circumstances, for example. If the average income of the families of the experimental group teenagers was higher, then these teenagers would probably have a better opportunity for adequate prenatal nutrition than the comparison group teenagers. Or the comparison hospital might serve older teens, or a higher percentage of married teens, or a higher percentage of teens attending a special school-based program for

Copyright © 2006. Lippincott Williams & Wilkins. *Study Guide to Accompany Essentials of Nursing Research*, by Denise F. Polit and Cheryl Tatano Beck.

pregnant students. None of these extraneous variables, which could affect the mother's health, has been controlled.

Another way in which the design was vulnerable to selection bias is the high refusal rate in the experimental group. Of the 217 eligible teenagers, half declined to participate in the special program. We cannot assume that the 109 girls who participated were a random sample of the eligible girls. Again, biases could be either positive or negative. A positive selection bias would be created if, for example, the teenagers who were the most motivated to have a healthy pregnancy selected themselves into the experimental group. A negative selection bias would result if the teenagers from the most disadvantaged households or from families offering little support elected to participate in the program. In the comparison group, hospital records were used primarily to collect the data, so this self-selection problem could not occur (except for refusals to answer the contraceptive questions 6 months postpartum).

The researcher could have taken a number of steps to either control selection biases or, at the least, estimate their direction and magnitude. The following are among the most critical extraneous variables: social class and family income; age; race and ethnicity; parity; participation in another pregnant teenager program; marital status; and prepregnancy experience with contraception (for the postpartum contraception outcome). The researcher should have attempted to gather information on these variables from experimental group and comparison group teenagers *and* from eligible teenagers in the experimental hospital who declined to participate in the program. To the extent that these groups were similar on these variables, credibility in the internal validity of the study would be enhanced. If sizable differences were observed, the researcher would at least know or suspect the direction of the biases and could factor that information into her interpretation and conclusions.

Had the researcher gathered information on the extraneous variables, another possibility would have been to match experimental and comparison group subjects on one or two variables, such as family income and age. Matching is not an ideal method of controlling extraneous variables; for one thing, matching on two variables would not equate the two groups in terms of the other extraneous variables. However, matching is preferable to doing nothing to control extraneous variation.

So far we have focused our attention on the research design, but other aspects of the study are also problematic. Let us consider the decision the researcher made about the population. The target population is not explicitly defined by the researcher, but we can infer that the target population is pregnant young women under age 20 who carry their infants to delivery. The accessible population is pregnant teenagers from one area in Chicago. Is it reasonable to assume that the accessible population is representative of the target population? No, it is not. It is likely that the accessible population is quite different with regard to health care, family intactness, and many other characteristics. The researcher should have more clearly discussed exactly who was the target population of this research.

Clinton would have done well, in fact, to delimit the target population; had she done so, it might have been possible to control some of the extraneous variables discussed previously. For example, Clinton could have established eligibility criteria that excluded multigravidas, very young teenagers (e.g., under age 15), or married teenagers. Such a specification would have limited the generalizability of the findings, but it would have enhanced the internal validity of the study because it probably would have increased the comparability of the experimental and comparison groups.

Copyright © 2006. Lippincott Williams & Wilkins. *Study Guide to Accompany Essentials of Nursing Research*, by Denise F. Polit and Cheryl Tatano Beck.

The sample was a sample of convenience, the least effective sampling design for a quantitative study. There is no way of knowing whether the sample represents the accessible and target populations. Although probability sampling likely was not feasible, the researcher might have improved her sampling design by using a quota sampling plan. For example, if the researcher knew that in the accessible population, half of the families received public assistance, then it might have been possible to enhance the representativeness of the samples by using a quota system to ensure that half of the research subjects came from welfare-dependent families.

Sample size is a difficult issue. Many of the reported results were in the hypothesized direction but were nonsignificant. When this is the case, the adequacy of the sample size is always suspect, as Clinton pointed out. Each group had about 100 subjects. In many cases, this sample size would be considered adequate, but in this case, it is not. One of the difficulties in testing the effectiveness of new interventions is that, generally, the experimental group is not being compared with a no-treatment group. Although the comparison group in this example was not getting the special program services, it cannot be assumed that this group was getting no services at all. Some comparison group members may have had ample prenatal care during which the health care staff may have provided much of the same information as was taught in the special program. The point is not that the new program was not needed but rather that unless an intervention is extremely powerful and innovative, the incremental improvement will typically be rather small. When relatively small effects are anticipated, the sample must be very large for differences to be statistically significant. Indeed, power analysis can be performed using the study findings. For example, a power analysis indicates that to detect a significant difference between the two groups with respect to one outcome—the incidence of toxemia—a sample of over 5000 pregnant teenagers would have been needed. Had the researcher done a power analysis before conducting the study, she might have realized the insufficiency of her sample for some of the outcomes and might have developed a different sampling plan or identified different outcome variables.

The third major methodologic decision concerns the measurement of the research variables. For the most part, the researcher did a good job in selecting objective, reliable, and valid outcome measures. Also, her operational definitions were clearly worded and unambiguous. Two comments are in order, however. First, it might have been better to operationalize two of the variables differently. Infant birth weight might have been more sensitively measured as actual weight (a ratio-level measurement) or as a three-level ordinal variable (<1500 grams; >1500 but <2500 grams; and >2500 grams) instead of as a dichotomous variable. The contraceptive variable could also have been operationalized to yield a more sensitive (i.e., more discriminating) measure. For example, rather than measuring contraceptive use as a dichotomy, Clinton could have measured frequency of using contraception (e.g., never, sometimes, usually, or always), effectiveness of the *type* of birth control used, or a combination of these two.

A second consideration is whether the outcome variables adequately captured the effects of program activities. It would have been more directly relevant to the intervention to capture group differences in, say, dietary practices during pregnancy than in infant birth weight. None of the outcome variables measured the effects of parenting education. In other words, Clinton could have added additional and more direct measures of the effectiveness of the intervention.

Copyright © 2006. Lippincott Williams & Wilkins. *Study Guide to Accompany Essentials of Nursing Research*, by Denise F. Polit and Cheryl Tatano Beck.

One other point about the methods should be made, and that relates to ethical consider- ations. The article does not specifically say that subjects were asked for their informed consent, but that does not necessarily mean that no written consent was obtained. It is quite likely that the experimental group subjects, when asked to volunteer for the special program, were advised about their participation in the study and asked to sign a consent form. But what about the control group subjects? The article implies that comparison group members were given no opportunity to decline participation and were not aware of having their birth outcomes used as data in the research. In some cases, this procedure is acceptable. For example, a hospital or clinic might agree to release patient information without the patients' consent if the release of such information is done anonymously—that is, if it can be provided in such a way that even the researcher does not know the identity of the patients. In the present study, however, it is clear that the names of the comparison subjects *were* given to the researcher because she had to contact the comparison group at 6 months postpartum to determine their contraceptive practices. Thus, this study does not appear to have adequately safeguarded the rights of the comparison group subjects.

In summary, the researcher appears not to have given the new program a particularly fair test. Clinton should have taken a number of steps to control extraneous variables and should have attempted to get a larger sample (even if this meant waiting for additional subjects to enroll in the program). In addition to concerns about the internal validity of the study, its generalizability is also questionable.

Results. Clinton did an adequate job of presenting the results of the study. The presentation was straightforward and succinct and was enhanced by the inclusion of a good table and figures. The style of this section was also appropriate: It was written objectively and was well-organized.

The statistical analyses were also reasonably well-done. The descriptive statistics (means and percentages) were appropriate for the level of measurement of the variables. The two types of inferential statistics used (the *t*-test and chi-squared test) were also appropriate, given the levels of measurement of the outcome variables. The results of these tests were efficiently presented in a single table. Of course, more powerful statistics could have been used to control extraneous variables (e.g., analysis of covariance). It appears, however, that the only extraneous variable that could have been controlled statistically was the subjects' ages; no data were apparently collected on other extraneous variables (social class, ethnicity, parity, and so on).

Discussion. Clinton's discussion section fails almost entirely to take the study's limitations into account in interpreting the data. The one exception is her acknowledgment that the sample size was too small. She seems unconcerned about the many threats to the internal or external validity of her research.

Clinton lays almost all the blame for the nonsignificant findings on the program rather than on the research methods. She feels that two aspects of the program should be changed: (1) recruitment of teenagers into the program earlier in their pregnancies and (2) strengthening program services. Both recommendations might be worth pursuing, but there is little in the data to suggest these modifications. With nonsignificant results such as those that predominated in this study, there are two possibilities to consider: (1)

Copyright © 2006. Lippincott Williams & Wilkins. *Study Guide to Accompany Essentials of Nursing Research*, by Denise F. Polit and Cheryl Tatano Beck.

the results are accurate—that is, the program is not effective for those outcomes examined (though it might be effective for other measures), and (2) the results are false—that is, the existing program is effective for the outcomes examined, but the tests failed to demonstrate it. Clinton concluded that the first possibility was correct and therefore recommended that the program be changed. Equally plausible is the possibility that the study methods were too weak to demonstrate the program's true effects.

We do not have enough information about the characteristics of the sample to conclude with certainty that there were substantial selection biases. We do, however, have a clue that selection biases were operative in a direction that would make the program look less effective than it actually is. Clinton noted in the beginning of the results section that the average age of the teenagers in the experimental group was 17.0, compared with 18.1 in the comparison group—a difference that was significant. Age is inversely related to positive labor and delivery outcomes; indeed, that is the basis for having a special program for teenaged mothers. Therefore, the experimental group's performance on the outcome measures was possibly depressed by the youth of that group. Had the two groups been equivalent in terms of age, the group differences might have been larger and could have reached levels of statistical significance. Other uncontrolled pretreatment differences could also have masked true treatment effects.

For the one significant outcome, we cannot rule out the possibility that a type I error was made—that is, that the null hypothesis was in fact true. Again, selection biases could have been operative. The experimental group might have contained many more girls who had preprogram experience with contraception; it might have contained more highly motivated teenagers, or more single teenagers, or more teenagers who had already had multiple pregnancies than the comparison group. There simply is no way of knowing whether the significant outcome reflects true program effects or merely initial group differences.

Aside from Clinton's disregard for the problems of internal validity, she overstepped the bounds of scholarly speculation. She assumed that the program *caused* contraceptive improvements: "The experimental program significantly increased the percentage of teenagers who used birth control. . . ." Worse yet, she went on to conclude that repeat pregnancies will be postponed in the experimental group, although she does not know whether the teenagers used an effective contraception, whether they used it all the time, or whether they used it correctly.

As another example of going beyond the data, Clinton became overly invested in the notion that teenagers need greater and earlier exposure to the program. It is not that her hypothesis has no merit; the problem is that she builds an elaborate rationale for program changes with no apparent empirical support. She probably had information on when in the pregnancy the teenagers entered the program, but that information was not shared with readers. Her argument about the need for more publicity on early screening would have had more clout if she had reported that most teenagers entered the program during the fourth month of their pregnancies or later. Additionally, she could have marshaled more evidence in support of her proposal if she had been able to show that earlier entry into the program was associated with better health outcomes. For example, she could have compared the outcomes of teenagers entering the program in the first, second, and third trimesters of their pregnancies.

In conclusion, the study has several positive features. As Clinton noted, there is some reason to be cautiously optimistic that the program *could* have some beneficial effects. How-

Copyright © 2006. Lippincott Williams & Wilkins. *Study Guide to Accompany Essentials of Nursing Research*, by Denise F. Polit and Cheryl Tatano Beck.

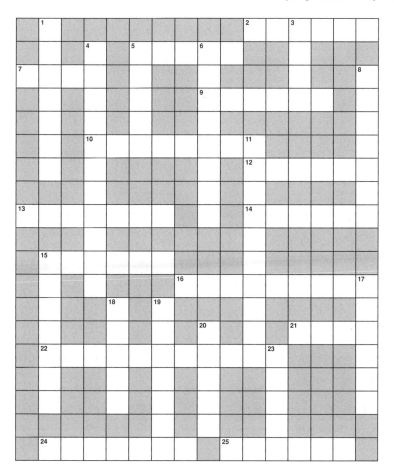

ever, the existing study is too seriously flawed to reach any conclusions, even tentatively. A replication with improved research methods clearly is needed to solve the research problem.

ACROSS

2. Quantitative results that are consistent with _____ are readily interpreted (abbr.).

5. A research hypothesis that is null is difficult to evaluate through standard statistical methods unless a(n) _____ analysis is performed.

7. Statistical procedures are designed to support rejection of the _____ hypothesis.

9. In critiquing the _____ dimension of a report, consumers evaluate the meaning that the researcher gave to the results (abbr.).

10. The most prestigious journals are _____.

Copyright © 2006. Lippincott Williams & Wilkins. *Study Guide to Accompany Essentials of Nursing Research*, by Denise F. Polit and Cheryl Tatano Beck.

12. One interpretive task is to suggest _____ of the findings for practice, theory, or future research (abbr.).

13. A _____ e prepared by students is usually a comprehensive analysis of a study's strengths and weaknesses.

14. A famous research principle is that _____ does not prove that one variable caused another (abbr.).

15. Reports submitted to journals are usually subjected to a critical _____ by other researchers.

16. The precept that correlation does not prove _____ is especially important in nonexperimental research.

21. A significant result is not necessarily of any _____ importance to practicing nurses (abbr.).

22. Researchers should take the _____ of their study into account when interpreting their findings.

24. Results that are _____ are especially difficult to interpret because of the possibility of a type II error (abbr.).

25. Before evaluating the meaning of results, researchers should evaluate whether they are _____ (believable) and accurate (abbr.).

DOWN

1. _____ editors usually solicit critiques of submitted manuscripts from researchers working in a similar area.

3. Researchers who evaluate journal submissions are called _____ reviewers.

4. In interpreting research findings, _____ explanations for the pattern of results should be considered.

5. Statistical support of hypotheses does not constitute _____ that the hypotheses are correct.

6. External and internal _____ should be brought to bear on the question of what study findings mean.

8. Evaluating the _____ dimension of a report concerns the adequacy of steps taken to safeguard participants.

Copyright © 2006. Lippincott Williams & Wilkins. *Study Guide to Accompany Essentials of Nursing Research*, by Denise F. Polit and Cheryl Tatano Beck.

11. Interpretations usually appear in the _____ section of a report.

15. Analysis of study data yields the _____.

17. Journals that do not solicit independent reviews of submitted manuscripts by other researchers (abbr.).

18. Reviews in which the reviewers do not know the researchers' identity, and vice versa.

19. The central interpretive task is to determine the _____ of the results.

20. When some hypotheses are supported and others are not, the results are _____.

23. In a comprehensive critique, the _____ and presentation of a report also come under scrutiny.

Copyright © 2006. Lippincott Williams & Wilkins. *Study Guide to Accompany Essentials of Nursing Research*, by Denise F. Polit and Cheryl Tatano Beck.

CHAPTER 18

Using Research in Evidence-Based Nursing Practice

■ A. Matching Exercises

1. *Match each of the statements in Set B with the appropriate phrase in Set A. Indicate the letter(s) corresponding to your response next to each of the statements in Set B.*

SET A

a. Research utilization (RU)

b. Evidence-based practice (EBP)

c. Neither RU nor EBP

d. Both RU and EBP

SET B   **RESPONSES**

1. Has been easily achieved in nursing   _____

2. Integrative reviews play a prominent role.   _____

3. Emphasis on translating knowledge to practical applications   _____

4. Integrates research findings with clinical expertise and client input   _____

5. Has given rise to several models by nurses   _____

6. Specifically begins with a knowledge-focused trigger   _____

7. The CURN project focused on this.   _____

8. Sackett and Cochrane were prominent proponents.   _____

■ B. Completion Exercises

Write the words or phrases that correctly complete the sentences below.

1. _____ is the type of research utilization in which there is an explicit effort to put study findings to practical use.

Copyright © 2006. Lippincott Williams & Wilkins. *Study Guide to Accompany Essentials of Nursing Research,* by Denise F. Polit and Cheryl Tatano Beck.

2. There has been considerable concern about the _____
   _____ between knowledge production and knowledge utilization.

3. The most well-known nursing research utilization project, conducted in Michigan,
   is the _____ Project.

4. _____ begins with an empirically derived
   innovation that gets examined for possible adoption in practice; _____
   _____ begins with a search for how best to solve specific practice problems.

5. The _____ Collaboration is an international
   effort to integrate and disseminate evidence about effective health care practices.

6. A(n) _____ ranks studies according to the
   strength of evidence they provide.

7. A widely held view is that the strongest evidence for EBP comes from _____
   _____.

8. The _____ model provides guidance
   for an individual utilization or EBP effort.

9. In the Iowa Model of EBP, the two starting points for an organizational utilization
   project are referred to as _____
   trigger and _____ trigger.

10. A typical method of assembling and evaluating evidence on a topic has been the
    preparation of a(n) _____.

11. Part of the RU/EBP process involves an assessment of the _____ of
    an innovation in a new practice setting (e.g., assessing transferability and feasibility,
    and computing a cost–benefit ratio).

12. Two methods of searching for prior research are the _____
    _____ approach (footnote chasing of cited studies) and the _____
    _____ approach (searching citations forward).

13. Meta-analysts sometimes conduct _____ analyses
    to determine whether the exclusion of low-quality studies alters the conclusions.

14. A well-established method of performing metasyntheses was developed by _____
    _____ and _____.

Copyright © 2006. Lippincott Williams & Wilkins. *Study Guide to Accompany Essentials
of Nursing Research*, by Denise F. Polit and Cheryl Tatano Beck.

■ C. Study Questions

1. Complete the crossword puzzle at the end of the chapter, which uses terms and concepts presented in Chapter 18. (Puzzles may be removed for easier viewing.)

2. Identify the factors in your own practice setting that you think facilitate or inhibit research utilization and evidence-based practice (or, in an educational setting, the factors that promote or inhibit a climate in which RU/EBP is valued).

_____

_____

_____

_____

3. Read either Brett's (1987) article regarding the adoption of 14 nursing innovations ("Use of nursing practice research findings," _Nursing Research, 36,_ 344–349) or the more recent (1990) replication study based on the same 14 innovations by Coyle and Sokop ("Innovation adoption behavior among nurses," _Nursing Research, 39,_ 176–180). For each of the 14 innovations, indicate whether you are aware of the findings, persuaded that the findings should be used, use the findings sometimes in a clinical situation, or use the findings always in a clinical situation.

1. _____

_____

2. _____

_____

3. _____

_____

4. _____

_____

5. _____

_____

6. _____

_____

7. _____

_____

Copyright © 2006. Lippincott Williams & Wilkins. _Study Guide to Accompany Essentials of Nursing Research,_ by Denise F. Polit and Cheryl Tatano Beck.

8. _____

_____

9. _____

_____

10. _____

_____

11. _____

_____

12. _____

_____

13. _____

_____

14. _____

_____

4. Read one of the following articles and identify the steps of the Iowa, Stetler, or Ottawa model that are represented in the RU/EBP projects described.

■ Fulmer, T., Mezey, M., Bottrell, M., Abraham, I., Sazant, J., Grossman, S., et al. (2002). Nurses Improving Care for Healthsystem Elders (NICHE): Using outcomes and benchmarks for evidence-based practice. *Geriatric Nursing, 23,* 121–127.

■ Robinson, C. B., Fritch, M., Hullett, L., Peterson, M. A., Siikena, S., Theuninck, L., et al. (2000). Development of a protocol to prevent opioid-induced constipation with cancer: A research utilization project. *Clinical Journal of Oncology Nursing, 4,* 79–84.

■ Samselle, C. M., Wyman, J. F., Thomas, K. K., Newman, D. K., Gray, M., Dougherty, M., et al. (2000). Continence for women: Evaluation of AWHONN's third research utilization project. *Journal of Obstetric, Gynecologic, and Neonatal Nursing, 29,* 9–17.

■ D. Application Exercises

1. Read the report on the meta-analysis by Taylor-Piliae and Froelicher ("Effectiveness of Tai Chi") in Appendix F. Then answer the following questions:

Copyright © 2006. Lippincott Williams & Wilkins. *Study Guide to Accompany Essentials of Nursing Research,* by Denise F. Polit and Cheryl Tatano Beck.

QUESTIONS OF FACT

a. How many of the studies included in this meta-analysis used an experimental or quasi-experimental design? How many were nonexperimental?

_____

_____

b. Did the researchers develop quality assessment scores for each study in the data set? If yes, how many study elements were appraised? What was the highest possible quality score? What was the average quality score for the studies used in the meta-analysis?

_____

_____

c. Did the researchers set a threshold for study quality as part of their inclusion criteria? If yes, what was it? Were any studies excluded because of a low quality rating?

_____

_____

d. The report indicates that the effect sizes were computed to compare aerobic capacity of subjects who had Tai Chi exercise and those who did not. What were the effect sizes weighted by?

_____

_____

e. How many subjects were there in total, in all studies combined?

_____

_____

f. Answer the following questions regarding information in Table 1:

■ What are the citations for the studies that used an experimental design?

_____

_____

■ How many subjects were in the 1998 study by Lan et al.?

_____

_____

Copyright © 2006. Lippincott Williams & Wilkins. *Study Guide to Accompany Essentials of Nursing Research,* by Denise F. Polit and Cheryl Tatano Beck.

■ In which study was the average age of subjects the lowest (i.e., youngest subjects, on average)?

_____

_____

■ What is the citation for the study that involved the briefest intervention?

_____

_____

■ What were the control conditions in these four studies?

_____

_____

■ In which study (and for which group) was the effect size the largest? Was this effect size statistically significant?

_____

_____

■ In which study (and for which group) was the effect size the smallest? Was this effect size statistically significant?

_____

_____

g. Answer the following questions regarding information in Table 2:

■ How many subjects were in the 1996 study by Lan et al.?

_____

_____

■ In which study was the average age of subjects in the Tai Chi group most different from subjects in the comparison group? What type of threat to internal validity does this suggest?

_____

_____

■ For which group of subjects, in which study, was aerobic capacity the greatest, on average?

_____

_____

Copyright © 2006. Lippincott Williams & Wilkins. *Study Guide to Accompany Essentials of Nursing Research*, by Denise F. Polit and Cheryl Tatano Beck.

■ In which study (and for which group) was the effect size the largest? Was this effect size statistically significant?

_____

_____

h. Were any subgroup analyses performed? If yes, were the subgroups based on methodologic features? Subject characteristics? Intervention characteristics?

_____

_____

i. Was the average effect size higher in the experimental or nonexperimental studies? Among men or women?

_____

_____

j. Did the researchers do a sensitivity analysis?

_____

_____

QUESTIONS FOR DISCUSSION

a. Was the size of the sample (studies and subjects) sufficiently large to draw conclusions about the overall effect of Tai Chi and about subgroup effects?

_____

_____

b. What other subgroups might have been interesting to examine (assuming there was sufficient information in the original studies)?

_____

_____

c. Did the researchers draw reasonable conclusions about the quality, quantity, and consistency of evidence?

_____

_____

2. Read the report on the metasynthesis by Beck ("Mothering Multiples") in Appendix G. Then answer the following questions:

Copyright © 2006. Lippincott Williams & Wilkins. _Study Guide to Accompany Essentials of Nursing Research_, by Denise F. Polit and Cheryl Tatano Beck.

QUESTIONS OF FACT

a. What system was used to conduct this metasynthesis? How many steps are in this process?

_____

_____

b. Were any of the studies in this metasynthesis grounded theory studies? Phenomenological studies? Ethnographies?

_____

_____

c. In how many of the studies in the metasynthesis was method triangulation used (Table 1)?

_____

_____

d. Which method of data collection was used in all six studies?

_____

_____

e. Which study in the metasynthesis obtained data from two parents?

_____

_____

f. How many study participants (mothers and fathers) were there in all of the studies combined?

_____

_____

g. How many shared themes were identified in this metasynthesis? What were those themes?

_____

_____

h. In Table 2, which theme was identified in all six studies included in the metasynthesis?

_____

_____

Copyright © 2006. Lippincott Williams & Wilkins. *Study Guide to Accompany Essentials of Nursing Research*, by Denise F. Polit and Cheryl Tatano Beck.

QUESTIONS FOR DISCUSSION

a. Was the size of the sample (studies and subjects) sufficiently large to conduct a meaningful metasynthesis? Did the diversity of the sample (in terms of participant characteristics and number of multiples) enhance the study or weaken it?

_____

_____

b. Did the analysis and integration appear reasonable and thorough?

_____

_____

c. Did Beck draw reasonable conclusions about the quality, quantity, and consistency of evidence?

_____

_____

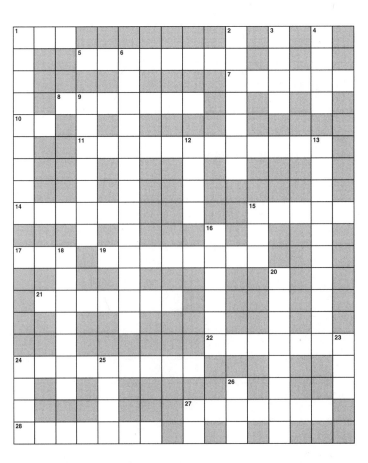

Copyright © 2006. Lippincott Williams & Wilkins. *Study Guide to Accompany Essentials of Nursing Research*, by Denise F. Polit and Cheryl Tatano Beck.

ACROSS

1. Practice based on best available evidence (acronym)
5. The medical school that developed an innovative clinical learning strategy in the 1990s
7. A model of RU/EBP developed by Canadian nurses
8. The originator of one of the earliest models of research utilization
10. The focus of the CURN project (acronym)
11. The type of utilization involving explicit attempts to base actions on research findings
14. The metric in meta-analyses is called the _____ size.
15. The evolving percolation of research ideas is called knowledge _____.
17. The U.S. agency that has issued evidence reports from its EBP centers is the A _____.
19. Momentum for an innovation builds through a process called _____ accretion.
21. A formidable _____ to RU/EBP is organizational resistance to change.
22. In the Iowa model, one path is through a knowledge-focused _____.
24. An important step in the RU/EBP process is to assess implementation _____.
27. One of the earliest projects aimed at improving RU was the _____ and Utilization of Research in Nursing (CURN) project.
28. A Canadian pioneer of evidence-based medicine

DOWN

1. Evidence-based practice involves combining research evidence with clinical _____.
2. One path in the Iowa model is _____-focused.
3. In many evidence hierarchies, the pinnacle is meta-analyses of _____ (acronym).
4. A well-established model of RU/EBP
6. Integration of qualitative studies
9. A stimulus for action in the Iowa Model
12. Research _____ has been conceptualized as occurring along a continuum in terms of specificity and concreteness of efforts (abbr.).
13. "Grey _____" refers to studies with limited distribution.
15. Another term for indirect research utilization is _____ utilization (abbr.).
16. The analog to instrumental utilization in Estabrooks' typology or RU

Copyright © 2006. Lippincott Williams & Wilkins. *Study Guide to Accompany Essentials of Nursing Research,* by Denise F. Polit and Cheryl Tatano Beck.

18. Integrative reviews increasingly involve formal _____ assessments of studies under review.

20. Meta-analysts are often interested in _____ effects to determine if interventions are equally effective for different types of people.

23. The stages of adoption in Brett's scheme are *awareness, persuasion, occasional use, and* _____ *use* (abbr.).

24. In Estabrooks' typology, _____ utilization involves using findings to convince others to make changes (abbr.).

25. According to research evidence, the ideal placement time for glass thermometers is _____ minutes.

26. One approach to searching for references, the _____ approach, involves "footnote chasing" (abbr.).

27. An international consortium that prepares and disseminates rigorous integrative reviews (acronym)

Copyright © 2006. Lippincott Williams & Wilkins. *Study Guide to Accompany Essentials of Nursing Research,* by Denise F. Polit and Cheryl Tatano Beck.

EFFICACY AND SAFETY OF SUCROSE FOR PROCEDURAL PAIN RELIEF IN PRETERM AND TERM NEONATES

Sharyn Gibbins • Bonnie Stevens • Ellen Hodnett • Janet Pinelli
Arne Ohlsson • Gerarda Darlington

- **Background:** Preterm and acutely ill term neonates who are hospitalized in a neonatal intensive care unit are subjected to multiple frequent invasive and painful procedures aimed at improving their outcome. Although several trials to determine the efficacy of sucrose for managing procedural pain in preterm and acutely ill term neonates have been developed, these have generally lacked methodological rigor and have not provided clinicians with clear practice guidelines.
- **Objectives:** To compare the efficacy and safety of three interventions for relieving procedural pain associated with heel lances in preterm and term neonates, and to explore the influence of contextual factors including sex, severity of illness, and prior painful procedures on pain responses.
- **Methods:** In a randomized controlled trial, 190 neonates were stratified by gestational age and then randomized to receive (a) sucrose and nonnutritive sucking ($n = 64$), (b) sucrose alone ($n = 62$), or (c) sterile water and nonnutritive sucking (control) ($n = 64$) to evaluate the efficacy (pain response as measured using the Premature Infant Pain Profile) (Stevens, Johnson, Petryshen, & Taddio, 1996) and safety (adverse events) following a scheduled heel lance during the first week of life. Stratification was used to control for the effects of age on pain response.
- **Results:** Significant differences in pain response existed among treatment groups ($F = 22.49$, $p < .001$), with the lowest mean Premature Infant Pain Profile scores in the sucrose and nonnutritive sucking group. Efficacy of sucrose following a heel lance was not affected by severity of illness, postnatal age, or number of painful procedures. Intervention group and sex explained 12% of the variance in Premature Infant Pain Profile scores.

Reprinted with permission from *Nursing Research* 2002; 51 [6]: 375–382.

Copyright © 2006. Lippincott Williams & Wilkins. *Study Guide to Accompany Essentials of Nursing Research*, by Denise F. Polit and Cheryl Tatano Beck.

Few adverse events occurred (*n* = 6), and none of them required medical or nursing interventions.

■ **Conclusions:** The combination of sucrose and nonnutritive sucking is the most efficacious intervention for single heel lances. Research on the effects of gestational age on the efficacy and safety of repeated doses of sucrose is required.

■ **Key Words:** neonates • nonnutritive sucking • pain • sucrose

Approximately 7–10% of neonates are born preterm (36 weeks gestation or less) and admitted to neonatal intensive care units (NICUs). Many full-term neonates are also hospitalized in NICUs for surgical or medical management of disease processes. Over the past decade, the technological and pharmacological advances in NICUs have increased the survival rates for these high-risk neonates (Philip, 1995). However, the incidence of painful tissue-damaging procedures to improve their survival has also increased. The ability of clinicians to effectively manage pain associated with these procedures has been greatly hindered by lack of high-quality evidence on the safety and efficacy of pain relieving strategies.

PAIN

Pain is defined by the International Association for the Study of Pain (IASP, 1979) as an unpleasant sensory and emotional experience associated with actual or potential tissue damage or described in terms of such damage. A recent "Note" has been added to the IASP definition that states that the inability to communicate in no way negates the possibility that an individual is experiencing pain and is in need of appropriate pain-relieving treatment. Therefore, the issue is no longer that neonates are incapable of pain according to the IASP definition but rather that they must rely on others to make inferences from behavioral and physiological indices for the assessment and management of pain.

The physiological responses to pain involve activation of the sympathetic nervous system (Stevens, 1993; Stevens, Johnston & Horton, 1994). The most common physiological pain responses for preterm and term neonates include: (a) increases in heart rate, respiratory rate, and intracranial pressure; (b) decreases in vagal tone and oxygen saturation; (c) changes in blood pressure; and (d) alterations in autonomic nervous system function (e.g., changes in skin color, nausea, vomiting, palmar sweating, and dilated pupils). These pain indicators have been widely studied in neonates; however, they may be difficult to interpret alone, as they can be influenced by nonpainful stimuli.

Behavioral responses to pain include facial expression, cry, and body movement. However, the quality of behaviors is dependent on gestational age and maturity. Preterm or acutely ill infants may lack sufficient energy to demonstrate body movements in response to pain. Their movements are less organized and less observable than healthy term infants (Craig, Whitfield, Grunau, Linton, & Hadjistavropoulos, 1993; Grunau, Holsti, Whitfield, & Ling, 2000; Johnston & Stevens, 1996). Similarly, cry characteristics may not be an appropriate indicator of pain in preterm or acutely ill neonates who are often unable or too immature to produce a robust cry. However, several studies have demonstrated that irrespective of gestational age, brow bulge, eye squeeze and nasolabial furrow are reliable indicators of pain (Stevens, 1993). Although preterm neonates are

Copyright © 2006. Lippincott Williams & Wilkins. *Study Guide to Accompany Essentials of Nursing Research,* by Denise F. Polit and Cheryl Tatano Beck.

less robust than their full-term counterparts, their facial expressions can be used as a valid measure of pain.

Significant hormonal and metabolic responses have been measured in fetuses (Giannakoulopoulos, Sepulveda, Pourtis, Glover, & Fisk, 1994; Teixeira, Fogliani, Giannakoulopoulos, Glover, & Fisk, 1996), and in preterm (Stevens & Johnston, 1994) and term (Anand, Phil, & Hickey, 1992; Kehlet, Brandt, & Rem, 1980; Porter, Wolf, & Miller, 1999) neonates. During painful procedures, these responses stimulate the release of "stress hormones" (e.g., catecholamines, corticosteroids, cortisol, growth hormones, glucagons, epinephrine, and norepinephrine) that increase heart rate and blood pressure, enhance liver and muscle glycogen breakdown, stimulate metabolic rate and improve mental activity (Anand & Hickey, 1987; Anand et al., 1992). Although these biochemical responses have shown an increase in preterm and term neonates in response to pain (Anand et al., 1992; Gunnar, Fisch & Korsvik, 1981), there are limited data on the normal ranges of these hormones, marked variability in the degree of changes between baseline and pain event, and difficulty in measuring these indicators in the clinical setting. In summary, neither physiological, behavioral, or biochemical indicators, when used alone, are valid, reliable, sensitive, or practical for identifying the existence, intensity, location, and impact of pain for a given population or situation (Stevens, 1993). Therefore, pain measurement from a multidimensional perspective appears to be the most appropriate approach.

SUCROSE

The administration of sucrose has been the most frequently studied nonpharmacological intervention for the relief of procedural pain in newborn infants. Sucrose is a sweet disaccharide consisting of fructose and glucose. The calming effect of sucrose is thought to influence endogenous opioid mediation, activated through taste receptors at the tip of the tongue, and nonopioid systems (Blass & Hoffmeyer, 1991). Indirect evidence for endogenous opioid mediation has been derived primarily through studies with animal models (Blass & Shide, 1994; Panksepp, Siviy & Normansell, 1986). Sucrose is altered in the presence of narcotic antagonists, effective with a short latency and effective after the painful stimulus has ceased.

Taste-induced analgesia in animal and human newborns is rapid, enduring, and dependent on the ability to detect sweet taste. Sucrose administered to preterm neonates via a nasogastric tube into the stomach failed to produce analgesia for heel lances compared to an oral route of sucrose administration (Ramenghi, Evans, & Levene, 1999). Sucrose is hydrolyzed into glucose and fructose through the intestinal epithelium that is present by 26 weeks gestation (Naqui, Biskinis, & Khattack, 1999). Given the rapid effects of intraoral sucrose, it is unlikely that hydrolysis in the small intestine is responsible for its pain relieving properties. Taste appears to mediate the opioid response.

Two systematic reviews (Stevens, Taddio, Ohlsson & Einarson, 1997; Stevens & Ohlsson, 1998) have addressed the efficacy of sucrose for procedural pain in neonates. Sucrose, in a wide range of dosages, was found to decrease individual physiologic and behavioral indicators of pain as well as pain assessed using multivariate composite indexes. However, there was inconsistency in the dose of sucrose that was effective, and

Copyright © 2006. Lippincott Williams & Wilkins. *Study Guide to Accompany Essentials of Nursing Research,* by Denise F. Polit and Cheryl Tatano Beck.

therefore, an optimal dose to be used in preterm and/or term infants for procedural pain relief could not be identified. Adverse effects were minimal with the use of sucrose, but the dose or administration method providing the smaller risk for less healthy preterm infants and very low-birth-weight infants is not known.

NONNUTRITIVE SUCKING

Nonnutritive sucking (NNS) is the provision of a pacifier or nonlactating nipple into a neonate's mouth to promote sucking behaviors without the provision of breast milk or formula as nutrition (Blass & Hoffmeyer, 1991; Campos, 1994; DiPietro, Cusson, O'Brien & Fox, 1994). Nonnutritive sucking has only recently been rigorously examined as a pain-relieving intervention. The calming effects of NNS have been observed in human and rat neonates, but the mechanisms underlying effectiveness remain unclear. They probably involve stimulation of orotactile and mechano receptors as a pacifier or nonlactating nipple is introduced into the infant's mouth. Unlike the mechanisms of sucrose, the orotactile-induced analgesia associated with NNS does not appear to be mediated through opioid pathways; it is not affected by the administration of narcotic antagonists, and its efficacy is terminated once sucking has ceased. Researchers have found that NNS reduces cry duration and heart rate during painful procedures (Campos, 1994). Although NNS has affected behavioral responses to pain, physiological responses including cortisol response, heart rate, vagal tone, or oxygen saturation (DiPietro et al., 1994) is not affected. Pinelli and Symington, (1998) examined the efficacy of NNS in a systematic review for many neonatal outcomes. Although preterm neonates who were provided with NNS during gavage feedings were discharged from hospital earlier, the review did not reveal any other benefits of NNS.

SUCROSE AND NONNUTRITIVE SUCKING

Researchers have examined the individual and combined effects of sucrose and NNS for pain-relieving interventions in term neonates (Blass & Ciaramitero, 1994; Allen, White & Walburn, 1996) Relative to sterile water, sucrose has been more effective in reducing behavioral pain responses. There is a trend towards lower pain scores with the combination of sucrose and NNS, but further research using larger sample sizes and composite measures of pain is required. One study (Stevens, Johnston, Franck, Petryshen, Jack, et al., 1999) examined the combined efficacy of sucrose and NNS for relieving procedural pain in preterm neonates ($n = 122$). Significant differences in pain responses (measured by PIPP scores [Stevens, Johnston, Petryshen & Taddio, 1996]) between the pacifier with water and control group ($F = 9.00$, $p < .003$), and pacifier with sucrose and control group ($F = 24.09$, $p < .0001$) were found. There was a trend towards lower PIPP scores with the sucrose and NNS group compared to the water and NNS group ($F = 3.62$, $p < .05$). Investigation of the efficacy of these interventions did not include more mature preterm or acutely ill neonates.

Although there is growing evidence that sucrose is effective in reducing pain responses, it is not clear whether the sucrose alone or a synergistic effect of sucrose with NNS is responsible. In addition, there is a paucity of data for preterm or acutely ill term neonates who may not tolerate larger volumes of a solution without side effects

Copyright © 2006. Lippincott Williams & Wilkins. *Study Guide to Accompany Essentials of Nursing Research*, by Denise F. Polit and Cheryl Tatano Beck.

(e.g., aspiration, bradycardia, tachycardia, or desaturations). Several studies (Johnston, Stremler, Horton, & Friedman, 1999; Johnston, Stremler, Stevens, & Horton, 1997; Stevens et al., 1999) have found that small doses of sucrose (0.012–0.12 g) reduce composite pain scores in neonates <34 weeks of gestation. However, further research on volume and dose-response for a wide range of neonates is justified. The main purpose of this study was to compare the efficacy and safety of 0.5 ml of 24% sucrose with a pacifier (NNS) with sucrose alone or sterile water and NNS for decreasing procedural pain associated with heel lances in preterm and term neonates. Due to the inclusion of preterm and acutely ill term neonates, the dose of sucrose was half the recommended dose from the meta-analysis (Stevens, Taddio, Ohlsson & Einarson, 1997). A secondary objective was to explore the influence of contextual factors including sex, severity of illness, postnatal age, and prior painful procedures on the efficacy of sucrose. These factors have influenced pain responses in previous studies. The Gate Control Theory (GCT) (Melzack & Wall, 1996), existing knowledge of the developing central nervous system (CNS), and data on factors that influence neonates' pain responses were used as explanatory models to examine effective pain management.

■ Methods

PARTICIPANTS AND SETTING

During a 16-month period in 1998–1999, 661 neonates from one university-affiliated metropolitan Level III NICU were eligible to participate in the study. Eligible neonates were born between 27 and 43 weeks gestation, <7 days of age, had 5-minute Apgar scores ≥7 or cord pH (arterial or venous) ≥7.0, and had not undergone surgery. Neonates were excluded from the study if they (a) had a diagnosed major congenital disorder (e.g., neuro-muscular disease, spinal cord injury), (b) had received analgesics or sedatives within 12 hours of enrollment, (c) had received paralytic agents (e.g., pancuronium) or (d) had parents who could not speak English. Neonates were not excluded if they required assisted ventilation, supplemental oxygen, or blood pressure support. Eligible neonates were stratified into three gestational age groups (a) 27–31 $^6/_7$ weeks, (b) 32–35 $^6/_7$ weeks, and (c) 36–43 weeks. Prognostic stratification for gestational age was used only to control for the effects of maturity at birth on the primary outcome, pain. Although other variables may have influenced PIPP scores, sufficient knowledge of neonates' pain responses based on developing neuroanatomy exist, and stratification for gestational age was a biologically plausible variable that may affect pain responses. Four hundred and fifty-two neonates were not recruited for the study (as their particular age stratum was full), parents of seven neonates refused participation (3%), and data for 12 neonates were lost to follow-up (due to equipment failure), leaving 190 neonates in the final sample. Of the 190 neonates enrolled in the study, no differences were found between those neonates who were not recruited, those whose parents refused participation, and those who were lost to follow-up.

The primary outcome of pain response, using the PIPP, was used to calculate the sample size. Using data from one prior study (Stevens et al., 1999), a reduction of 2 points on the PIPP score at 30 seconds following the painful procedure, (approximately 20% on mean observed scores) was considered clinically significant. A sample size of 186 (62 neonates per group) was required.

Copyright © 2006. Lippincott Williams & Wilkins. *Study Guide to Accompany Essentials of Nursing Research*, by Denise F. Polit and Cheryl Tatano Beck.

OUTCOME MEASURES

Efficacy. Efficacy was measured by assessing the infant's pain measured by a validated composite measure, the PIPP (Stevens et al., 1996). The PIPP was specifically developed for preterm neonates and term neonates, and includes the physiological, behavioral, and contextual indicators that have been the most consistent with neonates' pain responses across many research studies (Abu-Saad, Bours, Stevens et al., 1998; Stevens, et al. 1997; Stevens, Johnston, & Gibbins, 2000). The PIPP was derived from multiple data sets and has been shown to have face and content validity and evidence of beginning construct validity for preterm neonate pain measurement of various gestational ages (Ballantyne, Stevens, McAllister, Dionne, & Jack, 1999). In the PIPP, the physiological indicators of pain include the change from baseline in maximum *heart rate* and minimum *oxygen saturation*. The behavioral indicators of pain include the change from baseline in *brow bulge*, *eye squeeze*, and *naso-labial furrow*. The contextual indicators of pain include *behavioral state* at baseline and *gestational age* at the time of data collection. Indicators in the PIPP are numerically scored on a 4-point composite scale (0, 1, 2, 3) 30 seconds following an acute painful stimulus. Subsequent PIPP scores are obtained every 30 seconds by comparing changes from baseline physiological and behavioral indicators. The number of PIPP scores is dependent on the duration of the painful procedure. The higher the PIPP score, the greater the pain response. For all neonates, a score of <6 is considered minimal pain and a score >12 indicates moderate-to-severe pain (the range of scores is 0 to 21). Stevens et al. (1996) discuss instrument development and initial validation in more detail.

Safety. Safety was measured by determining the nature and incidence of adverse events, including: (a) choking, coughing, or vomiting following the administration of sucrose; (b) sustained tachycardia (heart rate > 200) or bradycardia (heart rate < 80) for >15 seconds following the administration of sucrose; (c) sustained tachypnea (respiratory rate > 80) or dyspnea (respiratory rate < 20) for >15 seconds following the administration of sucrose; or (d) sustained oxygen desaturation < 80% for >15 seconds following the administration of sucrose. The safety criteria were attached to each neonate's medical record and any adverse effects were recorded. A safety committee was established prior to study commencement. The members of the safety committee reviewed each adverse event, and rules for stopping the trial included severe choking or need for immediate medical intervention (e.g., intubation or resuscitation).

Severity of Illness. The Score for Neonatal Acute Physiology (SNAP: PE) was used as a measure of severity of neonatal illness. The SNAP: PE is comprised of indicators including birth weight, Apgar score at 5 minutes, and small for gestational age, as well as 26 items based on laboratory tests and vital signs. The SNAP: PE has been validated on over 27, 000 infants in 31 NICUs in Canada and the USA (Richardson, Corcoran, Excobar, & Lee, 2000) and has been used in previous studies using the PIPP.

Other Data. Other data such as the neonate's birth weight, sex, gestational age and frequency of prior painful procedures were obtained from the medical records. Data were collected prior to randomization and used to describe the representativeness of the study sample.

Copyright © 2006. Lippincott Williams & Wilkins. *Study Guide to Accompany Essentials of Nursing Research,* by Denise F. Polit and Cheryl Tatano Beck.

PROCEDURE

The efficacy of sucrose and NNS, sucrose alone, and water and NNS were compared in a randomized control trial using a centralized randomization table. Following ethical approval by the combined Research Ethics Board of the university and the university-affiliated institution, parental consent to participate in the study was sought. Once parental consent was obtained, the research pharmacist randomized neonates to one of the three intervention groups. All study solutions were prepared under sterile conditions, labeled as "study drug," and delivered to the neonates' bedside immediately prior to the scheduled heel lance. Based on the literature to support the use of sucrose and/or NNS, it was considered unethical to deny neonates a form of treatment. Therefore, sterile water and the provision of NNS were used for the control group. Because of the study design and intentional lack of a control group (i.e., sterile water alone or no treatment), blinding of the intervention was only possible for the two groups who received a pacifier. To minimize variation, the heel lance procedure was standardized by phases: (a) baseline, (b) intervention, (c) warming, (d) lance, (e) squeeze, and (f) return to baseline. In addition, one individual performed all but five (97%) of the heel lances. The stimulus (heel lance), procedure, and automated lancet were consistent throughout the study period; however, the use of pacifiers at other times in the NICU was not controlled for due to ethical consideration. The duration of the squeeze phase was dependent on the amount of blood required for the scheduled test, and hence not standardized across groups.

Neonates in the sucrose and NNS group received 0.5 ml of 24% sucrose via a syringe onto the anterior surface of the tongue followed immediately by the insertion of a Wee Soothie pacifier (Children's Medical Ventures, Inc., Weymouth, MA) into the mouth. The pacifier was held in place by the investigator or a research assistant as required 2 minutes before, during, and 5 minutes following the heel lance. The research assistant encouraged sucking by gentle, rhythmic motion of the pacifier, but data on ability to suck efficiently were not collected and may be considered a limitation in the present study. Neonates in the sucrose group received 0.5 ml of 24% sucrose via a syringe onto the anterior surface of the tongue 2 minutes prior to a heel lance. No pacifier was offered. Neonates in the sterile water and NNS group received the identical intervention as neonates randomized to the sucrose and NNS group with the exception of receiving 0.5 ml of sterile water instead of 24% sucrose. Neonates in each intervention group were positioned with their knees flexed towards their chest, arms close to midline and contained in a blanket to prevent large body movements. Only the foot to be used for the heel lance was accessible.

The physiological indicators of pain were recorded by using a SATMASTER™ data collection system ("EMG," Los Angeles, CA) that provides descriptive statistics for each phase of the heel lance procedure. Data were recorded by the SATMASTER™ system second-to-second and transmitted into a personal computer. The behavioral indicators of pain were recorded on videotape with a zoom lens (Sony digital zoom, handycam vision, 72X). Prior to the scheduled heel lance, the neonate's behavioral state, baseline heart rate, and oxygen saturation were recorded. An oxygen saturation monitor (Pulse Oximeter, Model N-3000, Hayward, CA) was applied to the neonate's hand or foot to record the heart rate and oxygen saturation. For each data collection session, the investigator calibrated the neonate's ECG monitor with the pulse oximeter

Copyright © 2006. Lippincott Williams & Wilkins. *Study Guide to Accompany Essentials of Nursing Research,* by Denise F. Polit and Cheryl Tatano Beck.

and the SATMASTER™ system. If there was a discrepancy in the recorded heart rates (>10 beats/minute) between the monitors (detected by the research assistant at the time of data collection), the data were collected manually by the research assistant using a preprinted and standardized form with 5-second time increments. Having the data collector enter a marker into the SATMASTER™ program simultaneously with a verbal command onto the videotape synchronized physiological and behavioral indicators.

Behavioral facial data were videotaped in real time, copied, and forwarded to a facial coder who had been specially trained in facial coding and who was kept uninformed to the purpose of the study, phases of the heel lance procedure, and group allocation (in the case of the two pacifier groups). An experienced coder did regular intrarater reliability and validity checks after approximately 25 neonates were randomized. The intra-rater reliability was high (alpha = 0.93). The research assistant who performed the heel lance procedure and collected data from the neonate's medical record did not know which solution the neonate was receiving with a pacifier.

The PIPP scores were manually computed from the raw physiological SATMASTER™ data and facial coding. The calculation of all PIPP scores were double-checked by two research assistants and double entered into a data management system by two separate research assistants blinded to group allocation. All data were verified for completeness. Logic checks were performed on the individual databases and there was a very low error rate in data entry (less than 1%). Manual calculation of physiological data (for discrepancies in heart rate between monitors) was required for eight neonates.

■ Results

Data were analyzed using the SPSS™ statistical package (Norusis, 1993). Representativeness of the sample was first determined by comparing data from the eligible refusers to those neonates who participated in the study. Later, comparing the study sample to the annual statistics from the study hospital's 1999 perinatal database determined representativeness of the sample. Neonates who were lost to follow up due to equipment failure recognized at the time of facial coding were compared to study participants and no differences were found. Demographic and other baseline variables were compared between treatment groups and descriptive statistics were calculated. There were no differences in any of the baseline variables. Data were then subjected to a repeated measures analysis of variance (RMANOVA), using the PIPP scores, to determine the efficacy of the treatment groups over time. The significance level for all tests was set at 0.05. To explore the influence of contextual factors on pain response, a hierarchical regression analysis was performed (Table 1).

RESULTS BY RESEARCH QUESTION

The Most Efficacious Method of Sucrose Delivery for Neonates Experiencing a Heel Lance. All neonates had a PIPP score at 30 seconds and 96% had PIPP scores at 60 seconds. Subsequent PIPP scores were not available because only 60% of the data were available at 90 seconds and 40% of the data were available at 120 seconds (as the

Copyright © 2006. Lippincott Williams & Wilkins. *Study Guide to Accompany Essentials of Nursing Research*, by Denise F. Polit and Cheryl Tatano Beck.

TABLE 1 Description of Sample Characteristics by Intervention Group

Characteristic	Sucrose & NNS (n = 64)	Sucrose (n = 62)	Water & NNS (n = 64)
GA (weeks)	33.69 (3.84)	33.9 (3.83)	33.67 (4.05)
Weight (g)	2207 (924)	2286 (1002)	2242 (943)
Age at enrollment (days)	3.12 (1.85)	3.02 (1.75)	2.67 (1.89)
SNAP: PE	4.14 (4.56)	4.68 (6.73)	4.00 (5.02)
Number of painful procedures	11.86 (2.21)	11.63 (2.3)	11.92 (1.56)
Duration of procedure (min)	11.13 (1.68)	10.68 (1.21)	10.92 (1.26)
Number of males	30 (47%)	32 (51%)	32 (50%)

Note. All values are expressed as means (*SD*) or percentages as indicated. NNS = nonnutritive sucking; GA = gestational age; SNAP: PE = severity of illness.

duration of procedure varied). The results are summarized in Table 2. A RM ANOVA was performed to determine the efficacy of the three interventions for reducing procedural pain. The pain scores (PIPP) at 30 and 60 seconds were used as the dependent variable. The between-subject factor was the intervention group and the within-subjects factor was time. There was a significant main effect of intervention group ($F = 22.49, p < .001$). There was no main effect of time and no interaction between treatment intervention and time ($F = 1.69, p < .12$). Post hoc analyses were performed to contrast the treatment interventions with each other. The PIPP scores were significantly lower in the sucrose and NNS compared to sucrose alone ($p < .002$) or sterile water and NNS ($p < .001$). No significant differences in PIPP scores between sucrose alone or sterile water and NNS groups were found ($p = .57$).

Determining the Nature and Incidence of Adverse Effects by Treatment Group. Due to the small number of adverse events ($n = 6$), only frequencies and percentages of adverse events by phase were calculated. Three neonates in the sucrose alone group desaturated during the study period, two neonates in the water and NNS group desaturated during

TABLE 2 Composite Pain Responses at 30 and 60 Seconds by Intervention Group

Intervention Group	Mean (*SD*) PIPP Score	
	30 seconds	*60 seconds*
Sucrose and NNS	8.16 (3.24) (n = 64)	8.78 (4.03) (n = 60)
Sucrose alone	9.77 (3.04) (n = 62)	11.20 (3.25) (n = 57)
Sterile water and NNS	10.19 (2.67) (n = 64)	11.20 (3.47) (n = 59)

Note. All values expressed as means (standard deviation); PIPP = Premature Infant Pain Profile; NNS = nonnutritive sucking.

Copyright © 2006. Lippincott Williams & Wilkins. *Study Guide to Accompany Essentials of Nursing Research*, by Denise F. Polit and Cheryl Tatano Beck.

the study period, and one neonate choked on the pacifier. No adverse events occurred with neonates randomized to the sucrose and NNS group. More adverse events occurred in the least mature neonates ($n = 4$) compared to the middle ($n = 1$) and most mature ($n = 1$) neonates.

Factors That Influence Pain Responses. A hierarchical multiple regression analysis was used to determine which variables contributed to the variance in the major outcome pain, as assessed by 30 second PIPP scores. Variables were entered sequentially into the model depending on the potential contribution to the variance in PIPP scores. The intervention group was entered first as contributing potential to the variance in PIPP scores. Neonatal characteristics that have been shown to influence pain response in previous studies (e.g., the number of painful procedures, post natal age, severity of illness, and sex) were entered last. Gestational age and behavioral state were not entered into the model, as they were contextual indicators used to compute the PIPP score. The intervention group explained 9% of the variance and sex explained 3% of the variance. All other variables were deleted from the final model, as they did not add information in the presence of sex and intervention group. There were associations between sex and PIPP scores, with male neonates scoring significantly higher PIPP scores than female neonates. The mean PIPP score for males was 9.73 (2.92) and 9.01 (3.25) for females; however, the differences were small and not clinically significant.

▪ Discussion

Although pain management for neonates has improved over the last few decades, many painful procedures such as heel lance continue to be performed on neonates without appropriate analgesia or comfort measures. The suboptimal management of pain is related to misconceptions and myths of neonates' capacity to detect, transmit, and interpret pain as well as concerns about safety of analgesics. Administration of analgesics to neonates requires careful consideration of the pharmacokinetics (movement of drugs in the body over time) and pharmacodynamics (doseresponse relationship) of the specific agent (Stevens, Johnson & Franck, 2000). In addition, developmental differences between the metabolic functions of preterm and term neonates' must be considered prior to the administration of analgesics. All neonates in this study received a form of pain management for heel lances. Heel lances were chosen because they are the most commonly performed painful procedure in the NICU. Sucrose was hypothesized to reduce pain by opioid mediation, activated by taste. The NNS was hypothesized to reduce pain by tactile mechanisms, while the combination of sucrose and NNS was hypothesized to offer the most efficacious pain relief.

Sucrose and NNS significantly reduced PIPP scores for heel lances in preterm and term neonates at 30 seconds. These results are generally consistent with comparative studies where differences in pain responses between term (Abad, Diaz, Domenech, Robayna, Rico et al., 1993; Haouari, Wood, Griffiths & Levene, 1995) and preterm

Copyright © 2006. Lippincott Williams & Wilkins. *Study Guide to Accompany Essentials of Nursing Research*, by Denise F. Polit and Cheryl Tatano Beck.

(Johnston et al., 1999; Stevens et al., 1999) neonates who received sucrose or water for pain associated with heel lances have been observed. The PIPP scores were also lowest in the sucrose and NNS group at 60 seconds; however, they generally increased from scores obtained at 30 seconds. As procedures become more invasive, as measured by duration of procedure and/or intensity of pain, the magnitude of physiological and behavioral responses increase. Porter et al. (1999) also reported that the magnitude of physiological and behavioral change is not affected by gestational age; neonates of all gestational ages can differentiate procedural invasiveness. Similarly, neonates of all gestational ages can demonstrate increased magnitude in response to increased duration (in seconds to minutes) of the procedure. These results are consistent with the present study. Although the present study did not have sufficient power to examine the influence of gestational age on the efficacy of sucrose, neonates in each gestational age stratum indicated a trend towards higher PIPP scores at 60 seconds, suggesting that the prolonged squeeze phase is more invasive than the lance phase. Further research comparing PIPP scores by gestational age over a longer duration of time is required.

A joint statement of the Fetus and Newborn Committee, Canadian Paediatric Society and the American Academy of Pediatrics has provided guidelines for pharmacological pain management in neonates. The administration of sucrose and pacifier are recommended approaches to pain relief for heel lances in preterm and term neonates. Sucrose and NNS are readily available in hospital nurseries, inexpensive, easily administered, and safe. In addition, the long history of use of sweet solutions and pacifiers for painful procedures further increase the likelihood of acceptance of sucrose and NNS as routine interventions for pain management in the NICU. Given the rapid and enduring effects of sucrose and NNS, they can be given together in advance of minor to moderate procedural pain. Although sucrose and NNS is not efficacious for moderate-to-severe pain, the combined therapy can be used as an adjunct with pharmacological interventions.

Other factors that have been shown to influence pain responses, such age at study session, severity of illness, or previous painful procedures were included in the present study; however, they did not appear to modulate pain responses. Sex explained some of the variance in PIPP scores, with male neonates having statistically but not clinically significant higher pain scores.

In summary, three treatment interventions were compared for the management of procedural pain in preterm and term neonates. The most efficacious and safe intervention was 0.5 ml 24% sucrose and NNS. Although there were a few adverse events during the study period, they were benign in nature, resolved spontaneously, and did not require medical or nursing intervention. In light of the relatively simple, yet efficacious, intervention to manage neonatal pain, changes in pain practice for selective painful procedures could easily be incorporated into standard NICU care. However, research on additional interventions that could be used in combination with sucrose and NNS is required in order to better reduce the pain associated with heel lances. In addition, the efficacy and safety of repeated doses of sucrose and NNS (alone or in combination with other interventions) for a variety of painful procedures is needed. Research is also needed on the management of pain for other high-risk neonates, such as preterm neonates less than 27 weeks gestation, cognitively impaired, or those with existing disease processes.

Copyright © 2006. Lippincott Williams & Wilkins. *Study Guide to Accompany Essentials of Nursing Research*, by Denise F. Polit and Cheryl Tatano Beck.

Sharyn Gibbins, RN, PhD, is Associate Professor, Faculty of Nursing, University of Toronto, Sunnybrook and Women's College Hospital, Toronto, The Hospital for Sick Children, Toronto, Ontario, Canada.
Bonnie Stevens, RN, PhD, is Professor, Faculty of Nursing and Medicine, University of Toronto, Signy Hildur Eaton Chair in Paediatric Nursing Research, The Hospital for Sick Children, Toronto, Ontario, Canada.
Ellen Hodnett, RN, PhD, is Professor, Faculty of Nursing, University of Toronto, Ontario, Canada.
Janet Pinelli, RN, DNS, is Professor, School of Nursing and Department of Pediatrics, McMaster University, Hamilton, Canada.
Arne Ohlsson, MD, MSc, is Professor, Faculty of Medicine, University of Toronto and Mount Sinai Hospital, Ontario, Canada.
Gerarda Darlington, PhD, is Professor, Department of Mathematics and Statistics, University of Guelph, Ontario, Canada.

Accepted for publication May 23, 2002.
The authors thank the Hospital for Sick Children, Toronto Ontario, Canada for the Research Training Award (Sharyn Gibbins, PhD, Sunnybrook & Women's College Health Sciences Centre, Toronto, Ontario, Canada) and the Ontario Ministry of Health, Toronto, Ontario, Canada for the Career Scientist Award (Bonnie Stevens, PhD, Hospital for Sick Children, Toronto, Ontario, Canada), and the staff and families at Sunnybrook & Women's College Health Sciences Centre, Toronto, Ontario, Canada.
Corresponding author: Sharyn Gibbins, RN, PhD, Sunnybrook & Women's College Health Sciences Centre, 76 Grenville Street, Room 445, Toronto, Ontario, Canada M5A 1B2 (e-mail: sharyn. gibbins@ swchsc.on.ca).

REFERENCES

Abad. F., Diaz, N. M., Domenech, E., Robayna, M., Rico, J., Arrecivita, A. et al. (1993). *Attenuation of pain-related behavior in neonates given oral sweet solutions.* 7th World Congress on Pain, Paris (Abstract).

Abu-Saad, H., Bours, G., Stevens, B. et al. (1998). Assessment of pain in the neonate. *Semin Perinatol, 22,* 402–416.

Allen, K., White, D., & Walburn, J. (1996). Sucrose as an analgesic agent for infants during immunization injections. *Archives of Pediatrics and Adolescent Medicine, 150,* 270–274.

Anand, K., & Hickey, P. R. (1987). Randomized trial of high-dose sufentanil aesthesia in neonates undergoing cardiac surgery: Effects on the metabolic stress response. *Anesthesiology, 67,* 502A.

Anand, K., Phil, D., & Hickey, P.R. (1992). Halothane-morphine compared with high-dose sufentanil for anesthesia and postoperative analgesia in neonatal cardiac surgery. *New England Journal of Medicine, 326,* 1–9.

Ballantyne, M., Stevens, B., McAllister, M., Dionne, D., & Jack, A. (1999). Validation of the premature infant pain profile in the clinical setting. *The Clinical Journal of Pain, 15,* 297–303.

Blass, E., & Ciaramitaro, V. (1994). A new look at some old mechanisms in human newborns: Taste and tactile determinants of state, affect and action. *Monographs of the Society for Research in Child Development, 59,* 1–80.

Blass, E. & Hoffmeyer, L. B. (1991). Sucrose as an analgesic for newborn infants. *Pediatrics, 87(2),* 215–220.

Campos, R. (1994) Rocking and pacifiers: Two comforting interventions for heelstick pain. *Research in Nursing and Health, 17(1),* 321–331.

Craig, K., Whitfield, M. F., Grunau, R. V., Linton, J., & Hadjistavropoulos, H. (1993). Pain in the preterm neonate: behavioral and physiological indices. *Pain, 52,* 287–299.

DiPietro, J. A., Cusson, R. M., O'Brien, M., & Fox, N. A. (1994). Behavioral and physiologic effects of nonnutritive sucking during gavage feeding in preterm infants. *Pediatric Research, 36(2),* 207–214.

Giannakoulopoulos, X., Sepulveda, W., Pourtis, P., Glover, V., & Fisk, N. M. (1994). Fetal plasma cortisol and B-endorphin response to intrauterine needling. *Lancet, 344,* 77–80.

Gibbins, S. & Stevens, B. (2001). Mechanisms of sucrose and nonnutritive sucking in procedural pain management in infants. *Pain Research & Management.* 6(1), 21–28.

Copyright © 2006. Lippincott Williams & Wilkins. *Study Guide to Accompany Essentials of Nursing Research,* by Denise F. Polit and Cheryl Tatano Beck.

Grunau, R., Holsti, L., Whitfield, M., & Ling, E. (2000). Are twitches, startles and body movements pain indicators in extremely low birth weight infants? *Clinical Journal of Pain, 16*(1), 37–45.

Gunnar, M., Fisch, R., & Korsvik, S. (1981). The effects of circumcision on serum cortisol and behavior. *Psychoneuroendocrinolgy, 6*, 269–275.

Haouari, N., Wood, C., Griffiths, G., & Levene, M. (1995). The analgesic effect of sucrose in full term infants: A randomized controlled trial. *British Medical Journal, 310*, 1498–1500.

Johnston, C. & Stevens, B. (1996). Experience in a neonatal intensive care unit affects pain response. *Pediatrics, 98*(5), 925–930.

Johnston, C., Stremler, R. L., Horton, L. J., & Friedman, A. (1999). Effect of repeated doses of sucrose during heel stick procedure in preterm neonates. *Biology of the Neonate, 75*, 160–166.

Johnston, C., Stremler, R. L., Stevens, B. J. & Horton, L. J. (1997). Effectiveness of oral sucrose and simulated rocking on pain response in preterm neonates. *Pain, 72*(1), 193–199.

Kehler, H., Brandt, M. & Rem, J. (1980). Role of neurogenic stimuli in mediating the endocrine-metabolic response to surgery. *Journal of Parenteral and Enteral Nutrition, 4*, 152–156.

Melzack, R., & Wall, P. (1996). Pain mechanisms: A new theory. A gate control system modulates sensory input from the skin before it evokes pain perception and response . . . reprinted with permission from *Science 150:971–979, 1965. Pain Forum, 5*(1), 3–11.

Naqui, M., Biskinis, E. & Khattack, I. (1999). Effects of 50% sucrose on pain responses in full-term male infants during circumcision. *Pediatric Academic Societies' annual meeting* (abstract)

Norusis, N. (1993). *SPSS for Windows: Base System User's Guide.* Release 6.0. Chicago: SPSS Inc.

Panksepp, J., Siviy, S. & Normansell, L. (1986). Brain opioids and social emotion. In M. Reite and T. Fields (Eds.), *The psychobiology of attachment and separation* (pp. 3–39). San Diego, CA. Academic Press.

Pinelli, J. & Symington, A. (1998) Non nutritive sucking in premature infants. In J. C. Sinclair, M. B. Bracken, R. S. Soll, J. D. Horbar (Eds.). *Neonatal Modules of the Cochrane Data Base of Systematic Reviews.* (Update February, 1998). Available in the Cochrane Library (Data base on disk and CD ROM). The Cochrane Collaboration; Issue 4, Oxford: Update Software; 1998. Updated quarterly.

Philip, A. G. S. (1995). Neonatal mortality rate: Is further improvement possible? *Journal of Pediatrics, 126*, 427–433.

Porter, F., Wolf, C., & Miller, P. (1999). Procedural pain in newborn infants: the influence of intensity and development. *Pediatrics, 104*(1), 313–19.

Ramenghi, E., & Levene, M (1999). Sucrose analgesia: Absorptive mechanism or taste perception? *Arch Dis Child Fetal Neonatal Ed, 80*, F146–F147.

Richardson, D., Corcoran, J., Escobar, G. & Lee, S. (2000). SNAP-II & SNAP: PE- newborn illness severity and mortality risk scores. *Journal of Pediatrics, 137*, 617–624.

Stevens, B. (1993). *Physiological and behavioral responses of premature infants to a tissue-damaging stimulus.* Unpublished doctoral dissertation, Montreal McGill University.

Stevens, B., & Johnston, C. (1994). Physiological responses of preterm infants to a painful stimulus *Nursing Research, 43*, 226–231.

Stevens, B., Johnston, C., & Franck, L. (2000). *The use of sucrose and pacifiers for managing neonatal pain: Are we alleviating pain or conditioning the infant.* Abstract #5. ISPP2000, the 5th international symposium on paediatric pain. London, UK.

Stevens, B., Johnston, C., & Gibbins, S. (2000). Pain assessment in neonates. In K. J. S. Anand, B. J. Stevens and P. J. McGrath (Eds), *Pain in neonates 2nd revised and enlarged edition* (pp. 101–135). Amsterdam: Elsevier Science B.V.

Stevens, B., Johnston, C. C., & Horton, L. (1994). Factors that influence the behavioral pain responses of premature infants. *Pain, 59*, 101–109.

Stevens, B., Johnston, C., Franck, L., Petryshen, P., Jack, A., & Foster, G. (1999). The efficacy of developmentally sensitive interventions and sucrose for relieving procedural pain in very low birth weight neonates. *Nursing Research 48*(1), 35–42.

Stevens, B., Johnston, C. C., Petryshen, P., & Taddio, A. (1996). Premature infant pain profile: development and initial validation. *Clinical Journal of Pain, 12*, 13–22.

Stevens, B., & Ohlsson, A. (1998). The efficacy of sucrose to reduce procedural pain in neonates as assessed by physiologic and/or behavioral outcomes. In J. C. Sinclair, M. B. Bracken, R. S. Soll, J. D. Horbar (Eds.). *Neonatal Modules of the Cochrane Data Base of Systematic Reviews.* (Updated

Copyright © 2006. Lippincott Williams & Wilkins. *Study Guide to Accompany Essentials of Nursing Research,* by Denise F. Polit and Cheryl Tatano Beck.

February, 1998). Available in the Cochrane Library (Data base on disk and CD ROM). The Cochrane Collaboration; Issue 2, Oxford: Update Software; 1998. Updated quarterly.

Stevens, B., Taddio, A., Ohlsson, A. & Einarson, T. (1997). The efficacy of sucrose for relieving procedural pain in neonates: A systematic review and meta-analysis. *Acta Paediatrica, 86,* 837–842.

Teixeira, J., Fogliani, R., Giannakoulopoulos, X., Glover, V., & Fisk, N. (1996). Fetal haemodynamic stress response to invasive procedures. *Lancet, 347,* 624.

Copyright © 2006. Lippincott Williams & Wilkins. *Study Guide to Accompany Essentials of Nursing Research,* by Denise F. Polit and Cheryl Tatano Beck.

A Theory of Taking Care of Oneself Grounded in Experiences of Homeless Youth

Lynn Rew

- **Background:** Homeless adolescents are vulnerable to poor health outcomes owing to the dangerous and stressful environments in which they live. Despite their vulnerability, many of them are motivated to engage in self-care behaviors.
- **Objective:** The specific aim of this study was to explore self-care attitudes and behaviors of homeless adolescents.
- **Method:** Individual interviews were conducted with 15 homeless adolescents. Interviews were audiotaped, transcribed verbatim, and analyzed using the constant comparative method of grounded theory.
- **Results:** Findings revealed a basic social process of taking care of oneself in a high-risk environment. This basic social process was supported by three categories: Becoming Aware of Oneself, Staying Alive With Limited Resources, and Handling One's Own Health, each including two processes.
- **Discussion:** Findings support Orem's conceptualizations of self-care and self-care agency and suggest the need for programs to support further healthy growth and development among homeless adolescents.
- **Key Words:** adolescence • grounded theory • homelessness

Homeless adolescents in the United States (US) comprise a population vulnerable to myriad health risks and adverse health outcomes. Numbering nearly two million, these youths include individuals who have run away from home, been removed from their homes by child protective authorities, or who have been thrown out of their homes by their parents (Shane, 1996). Living in the streets, abandoned buildings, cars, trucks, and public parks, these youths encounter environmental conditions that are both stressful

Reprinted with permission from *Nursing Research* 2003; 52 [4]: 234–241.

and hazardous to their health (van der Ploeg & Scholte, 1997). Despite their early childhood experiences and high-risk lifestyles, many homeless youths are characterized as resilient (Rew, Taylor-Seehafer, Thomas, & Yockey, 2001). Several studies have focused on the health-risk behaviors of homeless adolescents (Rew, Taylor-Seehafer, & Fitzgerald, 2001; Rotheram-Borus, Mahler, Koopman, & Langabeer, 1996; Sullivan, 1996; Yoder, Hoyt, & Whitbeck 1998), yet there is little known about the attitudes and behaviors that reflect their self-care and health-promoting behaviors. The purpose of this study was to develop a descriptive theory of self-care attitudes and practices grounded in the experiences of older youths who are homeless.

SELF-CARE PHILOSOPHY AND THEORY

The history of a self-care philosophy of health in the US can be traced back to the early to mid-1800s when Americans espoused their beliefs in personal responsibility for health and in having control over their own destiny (Steiger, & Lipson, 1985). The concept of self-care in nursing is generally attributed to Orem (1971; 2001), but it can be traced to Nightingale's (1859/1946) work a century earlier. Orem conceptualized self-care as "the personal care that human beings required each day and that may be modified by health state, environmental conditions, the effects of medical care, and other factors" (1985, p.19). Her conceptualizations led to the development of the theory of self-care deficits. Orem (1991) noted that self-care involved taking actions to regulate one's own functioning and development. She identified persons as self-care agents (2001) who (a) determined requirements for healthy functioning; (b) decided what needs must be met and how to meet them; (c) performed the needed actions; and (d) identified the outcomes of such actions. Conditioning factors (e.g., age, sociocultural orientation, patterns of living) affect a person's ability to engage in self-care (Orem, 2001).

Numerous studies of self-care have been done with children (McNabb, Quinn, Murphy, Thorp, & Cook, 1994; Moore, 1995; Rew, 1987), adolescents (Canty-Mitchell, 2001; Christian, D'Auria, & Fox, 1999; McCaleb, & Cull, 2000; Shilling, Grey, & Knafl, 2002), and adults (Leenerts, & Magilvy, 2000). However, few have explored this phenomenon in high-risk homeless adolescents.

HEALTH IN HOMELESS YOUTH

Homelessness is a highly stressful situation for most people (Craft-Rosenberg, Powell, Culp, & Iowa Homeless Research Team, 2000). By definition, homeless youths live in temporary quarters such as abandoned cars or buildings and have limited access to nutritional meals and healthcare services (Rew, 1996). Alcohol and other drugs are readily available among street people and this is a major health threat for adolescents who run away or are thrown out of their homes (Bailey, Camlin, & Ennett, 1998; Greene, Ennett, & Ringwalt, 1997; Koopman, Rosario, & Rotheram-Borus, 1994; Rew, Taylor-Seehafer, & Fitzgerald, 2001). Rew, Chambers, and Kulkarni (2002) conducted focus groups with homeless adolescents and found that these youths encountered numerous barriers in seeking healthcare services for symptoms of disease. These barriers included lack of available and/or accessible services, not knowing where to go, mistrust of healthcare providers, and inability to pay for care.

Copyright © 2006. Lippincott Williams & Wilkins. *Study Guide to Accompany Essentials of Nursing Research*, by Denise F. Polit and Cheryl Tatano Beck.

McCormack and MacIntosh (2001) conducted a grounded theory study of 11 home-less persons living in shelters and found that in spite of their homelessness, these persons were actively involved in promoting their health. The resulting theory focused on the concepts of person (who directs action), and health (the outcome of action that becomes the stimulus for further action). These researchers noted that pathways to health fol-lowed by this population began with accepting responsibility for self-care. Rew (2000) interviewed homeless youths and found that they used numerous strategies (e.g., making friends and keeping pets) to cope with the stress and loneliness that was part of their lifestyle.

Montgomery (1994) interviewed homeless women and identified a number of strengths among the participants, which included "stubborn pride," a positive orienta-tion to life, moral structure, stoic determination, and creation of self. It was argued that the social meaning of homelessness has a negative connotation but, nurses should recog-nize the many strengths of these individuals and advocate for social change that does not blame and further marginalize them.

It is well documented that homeless adolescents are vulnerable to poor health out-comes owing to the dangerous and stressful environments in which they live. Recent studies of homeless persons, including adolescents, suggest that despite the vulnerability associated with homelessness, many individuals display strengths that reflect their ability to engage in self-care behaviors. The purpose of this research was to explore self-care attitudes and behaviors of homeless youth.

■ Method

DESIGN

A grounded theory design (Strauss, & Corbin, 1994) was selected because of its poten-tial to address the patterns of behaviors within and between members of a particular social group (Strauss, & Corbin, 1998). Data were collected by individual interviews that were audiotaped and through observations of the participants recorded in field notes.

■ Participants

Theoretical sampling of homeless youths living temporarily in an urban area was used to insure a wide range of self-care experiences. Potential participants were recruited from youths seeking health and social services from a street outreach program (i.e., a clinic set up in a church basement) in central Texas. Criteria for inclusion were (a) 16–20 years of age, (b) ability to understand and speak English, (c) willingness to volunteer for an interview. This age group represented the majority of youths seeking services from this program. Fifteen youths (7 males, 6 females, and 2 transgendered) who were an aver-age of 18.8 years of age volunteered to participate. Saturation (sufficient or adequate data had been collected to meet the goal of the study) was reached at the end of 12 interviews;

Copyright © 2006. Lippincott Williams & Wilkins. *Study Guide to Accompany Essentials of Nursing Research*, by Denise F. Polit and Cheryl Tatano Beck.

TABLE 1 Participants in a Theory of Self-Care Grounded in Experiences of Homeless Youth

Pseudonym	Age	Sex	Ethnicity	Identifying Characteristics
Bev	18	F	White	Traveler; dropped out of school, has GED
Brett	20	M/T	Mulatto	Mother abandoned at age 14
Judi	19	F	White	Mother died when she was 16
Dawn	19	F	White	Traveler; smoking with family at age 11
Hal	18	M	White	Thrown out by family at age 16
Roy	20	M	Mixed	Abused by stepfather; disabled
Gene	20	M	White	Ran out of money in college; on his own
Cody	16	M	White	Used alcohol and marijuana at age 11 with father and brother; parents divorced
Chad	19	M	Latino	Wants to show parents he can be on his own
Liz	20	F	Mixed	Grew up in poverty; boyfriend committed suicide
Amber	18	F	Maltese	Wants to go to school for artists
Clarice	19	F	White	Traveler; looking for inspiration
Lee	19	M/T	White	Sexually abused by father; in foster care 8–18
Skip	19	M	Latino	Arrested at age 14 for stealing (not guilty)
Jerry	18	M	Native American	Emotionally and physically abused by parents

Note. F = female; M = male; M/T = male/transgendered.

three additional participants were recruited to verify the findings (Morse, 1998). These participants had been homeless for an average of 4.0 years. In the past year, the majority ($n = 13$) had lived in "squats," which are temporary campsites claimed by youths and other homeless persons. Demographic data and personal characteristics of these participants were summarized and pseudonyms were used to protect the identity of all participants (Table 1).

PROCEDURE

Prior to data collection, the investigator wrote down inital preconceptions, values, and beliefs about the population based on previous experiences with them and from a review of the literature. These initial ideas were held in abeyance until all data were collected and initial coding was done. The study protocol and consent forms were approved by the university Institutional Review Board for the protection of human subjects. The setting for the study was a street outreach program housed in the basement

Copyright © 2006. Lippincott Williams & Wilkins. *Study Guide to Accompany Essentials of Nursing Research*, by Denise F. Polit and Cheryl Tatano Beck.

of a church. Potential participants were told about the study by program personnel. Upon agreeing to participate, the youths were referred to the investigator who described the purpose of the study in greater detail and obtained written consent. Demographic data were collected by self-report, using a paper-pencil information form. Interviews were conducted either in a private area in the basement of the church or outside in a quiet courtyard area.

All interviews were tape-recorded with permission from the participants. Interviews lasted an average of 30 minutes and were guided by two main tour questions: (a) What helps you remain healthy living as you do? and (b) What would you like to tell me about how you take care of yourself? Upon completion of the interview, each participant received compensation of $10, a snack bar, and a beverage. The investigator also recorded field notes that detailed the youths' physical appearance and gestures during the interviews. Following each interview, the investigator's personal impressions of the participant and the participant's responses were written in a journal. This formed a portion of the audit trail, which was continued throughout the analyses as the conceptual development of the theory was documented (Morse, 1998).

DATA ANALYSIS

All interviews were transcribed verbatim by a professional transcriptionist. Confidentiality was maintained as (i.e., no names were used) during the interviews. The transcriptions yielded 193 pages of narrative data. Each transcribed interview was read and analyzed along with the accompanying field notes and journal entry prior to the next interview. The constant comparative method was used to develop open coding, analytic memos, and categories (Strauss & Corbin, 1994). To increase rigor in the initial coding process, the NUD*IST Q5 software program was used (Richards & Richards, 1998) to analyze the first eight interviews and verify initial codings. Coding from the software program was identical to the hands-on method used for the remainder of the study. To validate the interpretations of the data, member checks were conducted with three participants who agreed that the interpretations were accurate.

Each of the 15 interviews was analyzed line-by-line during (a) open coding, (b) the process of examining, (c) comparing, (d) conceptualizing, and (e) categorizing the data (Strauss & Corbin, 1994, p. 61). These initial codes used the language of the participants. Each interview was analyzed by comparing it to all previous interviews for preliminary conceptualizations. These early conceptualizations were recorded in analytic memos that were used in an iterative process of rereading and recoding. Axial coding produced categories in terms of causes, dimensions, and context. Twelve categories emerged and were diagrammed to indicate relationships between them. This resulted in the identification of some subcategories that were later clarified as processes of the three major categories. Continued refinement, including rereading the transcripts, rediagramming the concepts and categories, and returning to the literature, completed the process of analysis. Pseudonyms for the participants were used in analysis and presentation of findings.

Copyright © 2006. Lippincott Williams & Wilkins. *Study Guide to Accompany Essentials of Nursing Research,* by Denise F. Polit and Cheryl Tatano Beck.

■ Results

BASIC SOCIAL PROCESS

The basic social process, Taking Care of Oneself in a High-Risk Environment, linked the three categories together to form a descriptive theory of self-care for homeless/street youth. The three categories were: Becoming Aware of Oneself, Staying Alive with Limited Resources, and Handling One's Own Health. Each category contains two processes and several strategies (Figure 1). Taking care of oneself, self-care for homeless/street youths, is a process of deciding and acting in ways that enhance basic self-respect (caring about oneself) and that promote health. For the majority of street youths in this sample, this process begins with an awareness that life at home was intolerable and unhealthy and that they would have a better chance for survival and happiness if they were not living with parents or guardians. Many have had poor role models at home and learned to distrust "the system," represented by parents and institutions (e.g., schools, medical care agencies, child protective agencies). Most are more willing to listen to other youths from similar backgrounds (who they will find on the streets) than adults because in the past important adults in their lives have violated their trust.

Street life respresents freedom and a pathway to health and happiness for some youth. Given that many adolescents who live on the streets have made a conscious decision to leave an abusive or dysfunctional family, this avenue may be perceived as freedom from

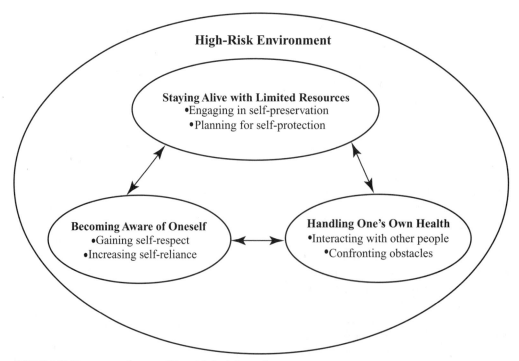

FIGURE 1. Taking care of oneself in a high-risk environment

Copyright © 2006. Lippincott Williams & Wilkins. *Study Guide to Accompany Essentials of Nursing Research*, by Denise F. Polit and Cheryl Tatano Beck.

the oppression and unhappiness they experienced at home. Brett said, "This is a learning experience. The streets are a stepping stone." This metaphor is supported by various experiences that youths have trying to figure out where they are going in life.

CATEGORY: BECOMING AWARE OF ONESELF

Self-awareness is a perception of oneself borne out of interactions with other people. Processes for attaining self-awareness are gaining self-respect and increasing self-reliance. Becoming aware of oneself begins with the adolescent's interactions with biologic and/or foster parents. Most of the youths in this sample described growing up in an environment that did not support healthy growth and development of children. Liz grew up in extreme poverty on an Indian reservation. "I didn't even really have shoes that fit, you know, I didn't really even have clothes. I'd be lucky if I got fed. My parents' idea of babysitting was to stick me in a closet with my brother and lock the closet until they come back." Lee, a 19-year-old transgendered youth, was sexually abused by his father who was also violent toward other family members. After his father locked Lee and his sister in a car, child protective services removed the children from their home and placed them in foster care. Lee ran away from this home because of conflict with the foster family about his sexual orientation. He spent some time in a shelter before entering the streets.

Brett, was sexually molested by his grandfather, enjoyed wearing his grandmother's clothing as a child, and was taken to a gay bar by his mother when he was 13. By the time he was 14, his mother had moved out of their apartment, abandoning him to take care of himself. His school grades plummeted and he had repeated psychiatric hospitalizations after faking suicide attempts, which he said were "for attention." He subsequently ran away from a hospital and remained on the street.

Out of such home-life situations, these adolescents grappled with a developing sense of self. Lee said, "I already knew who I was. I am in the wrong body—I am so in the wrong body." Amber also acknowledged her growing self-awareness when she said, in reference to a Mardi Gras party, "I'm like, no, you know, that's not me. Why would I want to do that [expose her breasts in public]?" Judi expressed her developing self-awareness related to interactions with her father: "Frankly, I'm more mature than him in a lot of ways . . . like in understanding human relations."

Developing a sense of self within families where the youth's sexual orientation led to conflict or where parents failed to provide mature care and guidance to the child led many of these youths to conclude that they were more capable of caring for and about themselves than their natural parents or those they encountered in foster homes. As Clarice put it, "I made my decision not to be around them [family]. I had to learn to build my self-confidence." Lee added, "I knew I could probably take care of myself pretty well."

Process: Gaining Self-Respect. After coming to the streets, these youths developed additional self-awareness through two processes: (a) gaining self-respect, and (b) increasing self-reliance. Gaining self-respect was reflected in the attitudes they expressed towards themselves and the strategies they used to stay alive and healthy on the streets. Brett philosophized, "I'm never truly going to be happy or find anybody if I have no respect for myself." Amber spoke of her practice of avoiding casual sexual encounters with

Copyright © 2006. Lippincott Williams & Wilkins. *Study Guide to Accompany Essentials of Nursing Research*, by Denise F. Polit and Cheryl Tatano Beck.

other street kids: "I respect myself more . . . I think it's [exhibitionism] so degrading." Lee spoke of defending his sexual orientation: "I'm not scared of no one [sic] . . . to an extent I'm very proud of myself because I've come a long way. I need to learn to respect myself and care for myself." This process of gaining self-respect contributed to a sense of healing from the brutal experiences of childhood.

Process: Increasing Self-Reliance. Increasing self-reliance was expressed as the tendency to trust one's own judgment and actions taken on one's own behalf above the judgment and caring actions of others. This process was expressed by all 15 of the participants. Many of these youths believed they could deal with any health problems encountered on the street with very little help from professional sources. Brett said, "I'm taking care of myself now better than I ever have in my life." Dawn, who knows she has anemia, said, "I, like, know what I have and how I'm supposed to deal with it." She, like several others, did not care to use prescribed medications (partly because the cost was prohibitive) or to pursue a more conventional lifestyle. Bev, who has asthma, added that she would not seek healthcare services for this chronic health problem unless it was very serious. She said, "If it's not life-threatening or anything, you're just going to be miserable . . . for a day or two . . . I mean, I don't want it [healthcare]." Roy and Judi described themselves as stubborn, saying, "I'm too stubborn to get treated for it" (Judi, speaking of her depression); and "I'm an independent person so I do it myself. I'm stubborn like that" (Roy).

Increasing self-reliance meant that these street youths such as Cody did not "wait for somebody to come do something for you." Strategies that increased their self-reliance included (a) taking care of a dog, (b) obtaining essentials without asking for help, (c) using natural remedies to treat cuts and upset stomachs, (d) improvising places to sleep and ways to travel, and (e) staying aware of their surroundings.

Despite their early experiences in homes that did not promote healthy growth and development, these street youths were becoming aware of themselves as agents of change. Most of the participants recognized unhealthy environments at home or in foster homes and relied on their abilities to protect themselves. By gaining self-respect and self-reliance through new experiences (e.g., taking care of themselves and their pets on the streets, traveling with friends, improvising to maintain their health), they were changing old patterns of feeling devalued and victimized into new patterns of feeling worthy and capable.

CATEGORY: STAYING ALIVE WITH LIMITED RESOURCES

Becoming more self-aware through gaining self-respect and increasing self-reliance led these participants to engage in daily self-care practices to promote and maintain their health. Living on the streets for these participants meant staying alive even though they had few resources such as regular meals, clean clothing, and a consistent place to sleep that would contribute to optimal growth and healthy development. However, these youths persevered toward their goal of finding a better way to live by meeting their own survival needs and protecting themselves from harm.

Process: Engaging in Self-Preservation. Engaging in self-preservation included strategies such as holding part-time jobs and panhandling ("flying a sign") to get food and getting

Copyright © 2006. Lippincott Williams & Wilkins. *Study Guide to Accompany Essentials of Nursing Research*, by Denise F. Polit and Cheryl Tatano Beck.

into fights to preserve one's dignity. Engaging in self-preservation was examplified in many commonsense self-care behaviors (e.g., eating fruits and vegetables instead of sweets or junk food, drinking plenty of water, getting lots of exercise [mostly walking], and staying clean). Most participants learned to care for their feet knowing that "boot rot" (tinnea pedis) would cause immobility. These youths also knew that sleeping restfully and staying out of inclement weather (rain and cold) were important strategies in staying alive and healthy, As Chad said, "This [living on the streets] really does take some work."

Process: Planning for Self-Protection. Aware that this environment was dangerous, youths described (a) having a dog for protection, (b) carrying weapons (usually a knife or chain), (c) staying with familiar people, (d) avoiding dark places and drug addicts, and (e) remaining cautious about the surroundings. Others were very specific about protecting themselves from sexually transmitted diseases by using condoms and getting immunizations for hepatitis B. Females, in particular, expressed an interest in learning more about self-defense. Clarice said, "I'm pretty good with self-defense and protecting myself—not making myself a potential victim."

There were diverse opinions about the topic of carrying weapons. Gene noted, "Several kids carry weapons. Some kids broadcast the fact they have these knives and these other types of weapons on them and I mean, that makes you actually afraid of what if these people do get drunk one of these nights?" Jerry added, "Nah [carry a knife?], some of my friends carry knives, but I figure I'd just get hurt more if I do that. I just stay away from dangerous situations." In describing how she protects herself on the streets, Liz said, "I've got my big huge dog and I know how to fight and I carry weapons [knife]." Bev also said, "Try not to go down dark places . . . if I'm by myself, show my knife. Yeah, I had a really big dog for a very long time—that was kind of my knife, I guess you could say. Nobody ever messed with me with him, you know."

By engaging in self-preservation activities and protecting themselves, participants showed how they persevered with limited resources. They were (a) highly motivated to survive, (b) knowledgeable of health and hygiene, and (c) resourceful in protecting their health and their lives.

CATEGORY: HANDLING ONE'S OWN HEALTH

Participants identified two major processes in handling their own health. These were interacting with other people and overcoming obstacles. Learning to handle one's own health was experienced through other people at home, at school, and in healthcare facilities as they were growing up. As independents, they become more aware of their knowledge about healthy behaviors and their lack of trust of authority figures and institutions. Judi claimed, "I'm very wary of Western medicine."

Process: Interacting With Other People. Participants were aware of healthcare resources available at the street outreach center where this study was conducted. Other people they met while on the streets or while obtaining services from the outreach center helped them to survive by giving them food and shelter. Traveling companions provided a safety net, a shield against loneliness. Clarice said, "I'm constantly around people so it's not so lonely." Interacting with peers as well as professionals became part of handling their own health.

Copyright © 2006. Lippincott Williams & Wilkins. *Study Guide to Accompany Essentials of Nursing Research*, by Denise F. Polit and Cheryl Tatano Beck.

Process: Confronting Obstacles. They identified a number of obstacles to taking care of themselves on the street. Many identified inconveniences in trying to find regular meals and a comfortable place to sleep. For example, Dawn said that although the street outreach program gave her cans of food, she could not cook: "It's hard enough to find a can opener." Clarice voiced her concern about adequate sleep: "Sometimes we sleep on real hard concrete . . . or the ground gets a little hard . . . so I get knots in my muscles." Chad stated, "You never really find like constant shelter. You never know where you're going to stay most of the time."

Lack of specific resources (e.g., telephones, transportation, money) prevented some participants from getting recommended follow-up care for injuries they had sustained while traveling (e.g., Bev broke both ankles jumping from a train).

The major obstacle to caring for oneself and staying healthy was expressed by Cody who said, "It's just hard to be out here on the streets and be sober. It's just that trying to handle my problems in a soberly manner is not easy. You get high together—that's basically how you establish friendships." Chad agreed, "That's pretty much what [using alcohol and drugs] everybody passes their time doing. It's a big problem." Hal and Roy thought the major obstacle to taking care of oneself on the street was that kids just "do stupid things that are unhealthy." Roy elaborated, "A lot of kids do a lot of very, very stupid things, I mean getting drunk . . . they don't know how to control like to slow down . . . and that can be very unhealthy for them."

▪ Discussion

Homeless youths described how they cared for themselves in an environment that was stressful and full of serious threats to their health and safety. For many, the decision to leave home came from experiences of abuse and neglect. These findings were similar to those of Leenerts and Magilvy (2000) who found that homeless women developed self-care attitudes and practices after first valuing and caring about themselves.

Becoming aware of oneself through the processes of gaining self-respect and increasing self-reliance support Orem's (2001) conceptualization of functioning with integrity and self-awareness as a criterion behavior for positive mental health. Statements from participants indicated that through these processes they were less fearful and felt both happier and healthier living on the streets than in their homes of origin. These findings are similar to those of Rew, Taylor-Seehafer, Thomas, and Yockey (2001) who found that homeless youths who perceived themselves as resilient exhibited less life-threatening behaviors than those who were not resilient. McCormack and MacIntosh (2001) also found that homeless individuals living in shelters had self-confidence and self-images that allowed them to speak for themselves and perform tasks to promote their health.

Staying alive with limited resources through the processes of engaging in self-preservation and planning for self-protection may be unique to the high-risk environments in which these participants lived. Previous studies of the influence of sociocultural factors on self-care practices in adolescents have focused on those living at home with biological parents and attending public schools (McCaleb, & Cull, 2000; McCaleb, & Edgil, 1994). However, many of the behaviors these participants described as self-preservation reflect

Copyright © 2006. Lippincott Williams & Wilkins. *Study Guide to Accompany Essentials of Nursing Research*, by Denise F. Polit and Cheryl Tatano Beck.

the universal self-care requisites identified by Orem (1985) such as maintaining sufficient intake of air, food, and water and preventing hazards. These self-care requisites have been measured in numerous studies of selfcare practices in household children and adolescents (Denyes, 1988; McCaleb, & Cull, 2000; McCaleb, & Edgil, 1994). Other behaviors such as carrying weapons would not be viewed as self-care strategies for the general population. However, given that these youths believe they have no protection other than themselves, it represents another type of caring for oneself.

Handling one's own health through the processes of interacting with other people and confronting obstacles supports Orem's (1985) conceptualization of self-care agency as the person taking action on their own behalf to "maintain life, health, and well-being" (p. 84). These findings also reflect some of the suggestions made by Ervin (1998) on teaching self-care to delinquent adolescents. Noting that learning to care for oneself is a critical step in developing independence in adolescence, Ervin adds that it is even more important for adolescents who lack family support. Homeless youth lack positive role models for self-care behaviors. Participants in this study recognized the simultaneous benefit and risk of interacting with others where alcohol and other drugs were the focus of social interactions, and led youths to do "dumb things" that compromised their health.

The majority of homeless adolescents had few positive role models and knowledge of self-care came from experience with their peers in the street environment.

Homeless adolescents who participated in this study are strong agents of self-care attitudes and behaviors. They have faced numerous adversities in their lives and have shown remarkable courage to redirect their lives toward healthy growth and development. Findings suggest that programs that support healthy growth and development in homeless youths are needed. Such programs can build on the self-care attitudes and behaviors the adolescents learned from taking care of themselves in a high-risk environment.

Lynn Rew, EdD, RNC, FAAN is Denton and Louise Cooley and Family Centennial Professor in Nursing, The University of Texas at Austin.

Accepted for publication February 10, 2003.
This study was supported by a research award from the American Holistic Nurses' Association.
The author thanks the staff and clients at Project PHASE, Austin, Texas, for their assistance and David Kahn, PhD, Associate Professor, and Sharon Horner, PhD, Associate Professor, School of Nursing at The University of Texas at Austin, for their invaluable consultations.
Corresponding author: Lynn Rew, EdD, RNC, FAAN, The University of Texas at Austin, 1700 Red River, Austin, TX 78701 (e-mail: ellerew@ mail.utexas.edu).

REFERENCES

Bailey, S. L., Camlin, C.S., Ennett, S. T. (1998). Substance use and risky sexual behavior among homeless and runaway youth. *Journal of Adolescent Health, 23,* 379–388.

Benson, P. L., & Pittman, K. J. (2001). *Trends in youth development: Visions, realities and challenges.* Boston: Kluwer Academic Publishers.

Canty-Mitchell, J. (2001). Life change events, hope, and self-care agency in inner-city adolescents. *Journal of Child and Adolescent Psychiatric Nursing, 14*(1), 18–31.

Christian, B.J., D'Auria, J.P., & Fox, L.C. (1999). Gaining freedom: Self-responsibility in adolescents with diabetes. *Pediatric Nursing, 25,* 255–260.

Copyright © 2006. Lippincott Williams & Wilkins. *Study Guide to Accompany Essentials of Nursing Research,* by Denise F. Polit and Cheryl Tatano Beck.

Craft-Rosenberg, M., Powell, S. R., Culp, K., & Iowa Homeless Research Team (2000). Health status and resources of rural homeless women and children. *Western Journal of Nursing Research, 22*, 863–878.

Ervin, M. H. (1998). Teaching self-care to delinquent adolescents. *Journal of Pediatric Health Care, 12* (1), 20–26.

Greene, J. M., Ennett, S. T., & Ringwalt, C. L. (1997). Substance use among runaway and homeless youth in three samples. *American Journal of Public Health, 87*, 229–235.

Koopman, C., Rosario, M., & Rotheram-Borus, M. J. (1994). Alcohol and drug use and sexual behaviors placing runaways at risk for HIV infection. *Addictive Behaviors, 19*, 95–103.

Leenerts, M. H., & Magilvy, J. K. (2000). Investing in self-care: A midrange theory of self-care grounded in the lived experience of low-income HIV-positive white women. *Advances in Nursing Science, 22*(3), 58–75.

McCaleb, A., & Cull, V. V. (2000). Sociocultural influences and self-care practices of middle adolescents. *Journal of Pediatric Nursing, 15*(1), 30–35.

McCormack, D., & MacIntosh, J. (2001). Research with homeless people uncovers a model of health. *Western Journal of Nursing Research, 23*, 679–697.

McNabb, W. L., Quinn, M. T., Murphy, D. M., Thorp, F. K., & Cook, S. (1994). Increasing children's responsibility for diabetes self-care: The In Control study. *Diabetes Educator, 20*, 121–124.

Montogomery, C. (1994). Swimming upstream: The strengths of women who survive homelessness. *Advances in Nursing Science, 16*(3), 34–45.

Moore, J. B. (1995). Measuring the self-care practice of children and adolescents: Instrument development. *Maternal-Child Nursing Journal, 23*(3), 101–108.

Morse, J. M. (1998) Designing funded qualitative research. In N. K. Denzin, & Y. S. Lincoln (Eds.). *Strategies of qualitative inquiry* (pp. 56–85). Thousand Oaks, CA: Sage Publications.

Nightingale, F. (1859/1946). *Notes on nursing: What it is, and what it is not.* London: Harrison and Sons.

Orem, D. E. (1971). *Nursing: Concepts of practice.* New York: McGraw-Hill Book Company.

Orem, D. E. (2001). *Nursing: Concepts of practice* (6th ed.). St. Louis: Mosby.

Rew, L. (1987). The relationship between self-care behaviors and selected psychosocial variables in children with asthma. *Journal of Pediatric Nursing, 2*, 333–341.

Rew, L. (1996). Health risks of homeless adolescents: Implications for holistic nursing. *Journal of Holistic Nursing, 14*, 348–359.

Rew, L, (2000). Friends and pets as companions: Strategies for coping with loneliness among homeless youth, *Journal of Child and Adolescent Psychiatric Nursing, 13*, 125–140.

Rew, L., Chambers, K. B., & Kulkarni, S. (2002). Planning a sexual health promotion intervention with homeless adolescents. *Nursing Research, 51*, 168–174.

Rew, L., Taylor-Seehafer, M., & Fitzgerald, M. L.(2001). Sexual abuse, alcohol and other drug use, and suicidal behaviors in homeless adolescents. *Issues in Comprehensive Pediatric Nursing, 24*, 225–240.

Rew, L., Taylor-Seehafer, M., Thomas, N. Y., & Yockey, R. D. (2001). Correlates of resilience in homeless adolescents. *Journal of Nursing Scholarship, 33*(1), 33–40.

Richards, T.J., & Richards, I. (1998). Using computers in qualitative research. In N. K. Denzin, & Y. S. Lincoln (Eds.). *Collecting and interpreting qualitative materials.* Thousand Oaks, CA: Sage Publishers.

Rotheram-Borus, M. J., Mahler, K. A., Koopman. C., & Langabeer, K. (1996). Sexual abuse history and associated multiple risk behavior in adolescent runaways. *American Journal of Orthopsychiatry, 66*, 390–400.

Shilling, L. S., Grey, M., & Knafl, K. (2002). The concept of self-management of type 1 diabetes in children and adolescents: An evolutionary concept analysis. *Journal of Advanced Nursing, 37*(1), 87–99.

Steiger, N. J., & Lipson, J. G. (1985). *Self-care nursing theory and practice.* Bowie, MD: Brady Communications Company, Inc.

Strauss, A., Corbin, J. (1994). *Basics of qualitative research; Grounded theory procedures and techniques.* Newbury Park: Sage publications.

Strauss, A., & Corbin, J. (1998). Grounded theory methodology. In N. K. Denzin, & Y. S. Lincoln (Eds.). *Strategies of qualitative inquiry* (pp. 158–183). Thousand Oaks, CA: Sage Publications.

Sullivan, T. R. (1996). The challenge of HIV prevention among high-risk adolescents. *Health & Social Work, 21*(1), 58–65.

Yoder, K. A., Hoyt., D. R., & Whitbeck, L. B. (1998). Suicidal behavior among homeless and runaway adolescents. *Journal of Youth & Adolescence, 27*, 753–771.

Copyright © 2006. Lippincott Williams & Wilkins. *Study Guide to Accompany Essentials of Nursing Research,* by Denise F. Polit and Cheryl Tatano Beck.

OLDER MEN'S HEALTH

Motivation, Self-Ratings, and Behaviors

Susan J. Loeb

- **Background**: There is a documented need to examine the complex motivational systems that lead individuals to adopt health-promoting behaviors and to evaluate the psychosocial aspects of male health. A study focused on health motivation as a determinant of self-rated health and health behaviors among older men was therefore undertaken.
- **Objectives**: This study aimed to explore the relations among health motivation, self-rated health, and health behaviors in community-dwelling older men.
- **Methods**: A descriptive, correlational survey design was used for this study of 135 community-dwelling men ages 55 years and older. The questionnaire packet included a demographic tool, the Older Men's Health Program and Screening Inventory, the Health-Promotion Activities of Older Adults Measure, and the Health Self-Determinism Index.
- **Results**: Older men with more intrinsic motivation rated their health as better ($p \leq .001$) and assessed their lifestyles as more healthy ($p \leq .001$) than did their counterparts with more extrinsic motivation. Whereas anticipated benefits (a potential motivator) were significantly related to health-promoting behaviors ($p \leq .001$), health program attendance ($p \leq .001$), and health screening participation ($p \leq .01$), the Health Self-Determinism Index score did not demonstrate significant relations with any of these three variables.
- **Conclusions**: The findings suggest that promoting self-motivation may be key to increasing older men's perceptions of health and well-being. Further exploration of anticipated benefits as a motivator of health-promotion activities is warranted, as well as intervention studies to promote older men's health screening and program attendance.
- **Key Words**: health-promoting behaviors • motivation • older men • self-rated health

The achievement and maintenance of higher well-being levels hold promise as ways for older adults, many of whom have limited incomes, to combat the ever-increasing cost of medical care and work toward the attainment of optimal health. Watson and Pulliam (2000) suggested that increasing older adults' well-being will serve not only to improve

Reprinted with permission from *Nursing Research* 2004; 53 [3]: 198–206.

Copyright © 2006. Lippincott Williams & Wilkins. *Study Guide to Accompany Essentials of Nursing Research*, by Denise F. Polit and Cheryl Tatano Beck.

their quality of life and protect their financial resources, but also to decrease our nation's yearly healthcare costs significantly. Increased attention must be directed toward promoting the health of elders if an increase in healthy years is to be achieved rather than merely prolonged life expectancy (Minkler, Schauffler, & Clements-Nolle, 2000). Specifically, there is a need for more applied research addressing motivational strategies designed to increase participation in health-promotion activities, particularly by older men (Loeb, O'Neill, & Gueldner, 2001).

Elderly men are a population of extraordinary concern because males reportedly value health less (Felton, Parsons, & Bartoces, 1997), participate in fewer health screenings (Zabalegui, 1994), experience poorer health, have shorter life expectancies, and allow an illness to progress longer before consulting with a doctor than their female counterparts (Baker, 2001). Despite the clear necessity for addressing challenges to older men's health, elderly men have been described as both a forgotten minority (Kosberg & Kaye, 1997) and invisible in gerontology (Kosberg & Mangum, 2002). This concerning phenomenon may be attributed to older men's smaller numbers, their lack of advocacy by gerontologic organizations, and the mistaken perception that older men experience a better quality of life than older women (Kosberg & Mangum, 2002). It is important to include older men of diverse ethnic and cultural backgrounds in studies because prevalence of health conditions, risk factors for diseases, and factors impacting health may vary across individuals of different races, ethnicities, and cultures (Wrobel & Shapiro, 1999). A factor contributing to diversity in a population is geographic location of residence. Thus, efforts to include participants from both rural and urban areas are essential. Krout, McCulloch, and Kivett (1997) assert that few researchers actually have focused on comparing rural and urban older males.

In response to the need for research addressing older men's health, the current study focuses exclusively on elderly men. Additionally, this research represents an extension of prior investigations because a variety of health behaviors are explored simultaneously (i.e. health-promotion activities, health screening participation, and formal health-promotion program participation) and a variety of self-ratings of health are included.

■ Motivation and Attitudes in Relation to Healthy Behaviors

Earlier, Rosenstock (1960) reviewed the findings of studies within the disciplines of the social sciences to address determinants of individuals' participation in public health programs. However, the motivating factors for health-promoting behaviors among elderly individuals remain uncertain and may differ from those of middle-aged and young adults (Miller & Iris, 2002). In their focus group study of 45 older men and women, Miller and Iris (2002) found that motivators for health behaviors included a desire to feel better, gain social support and combat loneliness, substitute a positive health behavior for a prior negative behavior (i.e., drinking alcohol), take on a challenge (especially related to participation in physical activities), and continue with lifelong positive health habits. A supportive spouse was reported to be an especially important motivator for the older men in the study. Similarly, a focus group study of 37 community-dwelling elders living

Copyright © 2006. Lippincott Williams & Wilkins. *Study Guide to Accompany Essentials of Nursing Research,* by Denise F. Polit and Cheryl Tatano Beck.

with multiple chronic health conditions found social support to be key in long-term adherence to an exercise program (Loeb, Penrod, Falkenstern, Gueldner, & Poon, 2003).

Frenn's (1996) grounded theory study investigating elder's perceptions of health behaviors identified two constructs of intrinsic motivation as important for health promotion: self-determination and perceived competence. Furthermore, the participants identified external forces, the way they were raised, and new awareness as important aspects of motivation for healthy behaviors. Haq and Griffin's (1996) survey of 156 elders found that more intrinsic health motivation was related to better health and greater participation in health-promoting behaviors. Also, interpersonal relationships and greater physical activity have been found to be significantly and positively related to more intrinsic health motivation (Lucas, Orshan, & Cook, 2000). Finally, a qualitative study (Gabhainn et al., 1999) explored sociodemographic variations in perspectives on cardiovascular disease. Older men were the least motivated for health behavior modifications and expressed an attitude that they were too old to change. In light of prior study findings, increased insights about how health motivation relates to various health behaviors in elderly males would guide nurses in planning health programs that better meet older men's needs.

▪ Self-Rated Health

The early work of Maddox (1962) warned that self-rated health and physician-rated health may not be identical. However, more recently it has been established that elders' self-reports of health status are reliable indicators, as demonstrated through associations with objective measures of health (Riffle, Yoho, & Sams, 1989), and that these self-reports have significant relations with functional ability and numbers of prescription drugs (Idler & Kasl, 1995). Self-rated health also is useful for ascertaining patterns before and after sentinel health events (Diehr, Williamson, Patrick, Bild, & Burke, 2001). Borawski, Kinney, and Kahana (1996) reviewed a number of well-designed epidemiologic studies, all of which found a robust relation between self-rated health and mortality, even after control was used for a wide variety of potentially confounding variables.

▪ Health Behaviors

Padula (1997a) indicated that health behaviors to be explored in older adults include attendance at formal health-promotion programs, participation in health screenings, and the following variety of health-promotion activities: exercising, avoiding health hazards, promoting one's safety, visiting healthcare providers on a regular basis, eating healthy foods, limiting alcohol intake, managing stress, seeking out health information, and ensuring adequate sleep and rest. Participation in such health behaviors is a means by which older men strive to meet the *Healthy People 2010* goal of increasing years of functional health (U. S. Department of Health and Human Services [USDHHS], 2001).

Copyright © 2006. Lippincott Williams & Wilkins. *Study Guide to Accompany Essentials of Nursing Research*, by Denise F. Polit and Cheryl Tatano Beck.

▪ Theoretical Framework

The Health-Promoting Self-Care System Model was the conceptual framework chosen to guide this study because it links nursing with both the attitudinal and behavioral patterns of clients' health (Simmons, 1990) (Figure 1). This model synthesizes and expands upon facets of the Health Promotion Model (Pender, 1987), the Interaction Model of

Basic conditioning factors
    Demographics
    Environmental influences
    Perceived health status

Self-care requisites
    Universal
    Developmental

Therapeutic self-care demand

Exercise of self-care agency
    Motivation
    Values

Health-promoting self-care
    Health responsibility
    Exercise
    Nutrition
    Stress management

Health outcomes
    Satisfaction with health-promoting self-care

FIGURE 1. From The Health-Promoting Self-Care System Model: Directions for nursing research and practice by S. J. Simmons, 1990, *Journal of Advanced Nursing, 15*, 1164. Copyright 1990 by Blackwell Science. Adapted with permission.

Copyright © 2006. Lippincott Williams & Wilkins. *Study Guide to Accompany Essentials of Nursing Research*, by Denise F. Polit and Cheryl Tatano Beck.

Client Health Behavior (Cox, 1982), and the Self-Care Deficit Nursing Theory (Orem, 1985). Simmons' (1990) model is based on the principles that health responsibility and self-care are central to health promotion and that people are able to gain the attitudes, knowledge, and skills necessary for participation in health-promoting behaviors. Finally, the model is useful for explicating the patterns among factors influencing health-promoting lifestyles (Simmons, 1990). Considering this model, the purpose of this study was to explore the relations among health motivation, self-ratings of health, and various health behaviors in a sample of community-dwelling older men.

■ Methods

SETTINGS AND SAMPLE

A convenience sample of older men were accessed at a "55-Alive" drivers' safety class held at a hospital, senior exercise classes that met in a church community room, seven senior citizen centers (5 rural and 2 urban), two McDonald's restaurants (only one yielded participants), and social groups of older men known by the investigator (i.e., neighbors and friends). Recruitment took place in both urban and rural regions of a Mid-Atlantic state to achieve a more ethnically diverse sample, because in that state, 97.9% of the rural dwellers are White (U. S. Census Bureau, 2000). In particular, urban recruitment sites facilitated access to more African American older men ($n = 25$, 18.5%). However, more elderly men were accessed from the rural locations (61%) because of greater success in gaining permission from the agencies/businesses. A rural McDonald's provided the researcher with almost as many participants ($n = 34$, 25.2%) as the second and third most participatory sites combined (an urban exercise class and an urban senior center yielding 19 and 16 participants, respectively), which was not surprising because McDonald's has targeted older men via television marketing (Bone, 1991). Convenience sampling was chosen because it is well suited for community settings, where limited space, time for recruitment, and data collection procedures are challenges.

The inclusion criteria for this study were the male gender; age of 55 years or older; ability to read, understand, and write English; and absence of obvious cognitive impairments. Originally, 139 men agreed to participate. However, two questionnaires were excluded because of unacceptable amounts of missing data, and two other men excused themselves and never returned, resulting in a total of 135 participants.

Power was computed for regression analysis, the most sophisticated level of statistics. Therefore, the conventional standards of .05 for committing a Type 1 error (alpha) and .20 for committing a Type 2 error (beta), as well as an effect size of .10, which Cohen (1988) identified as a small to moderate effect size for regression analysis, were chosen, resulting in a minimum sample size of 130 participants needed to achieve a power level of .80.

DESIGN AND PROCEDURES

A descriptive, correlational survey design was used. Approval for research involving human subjects was obtained through the office for regulatory compliance at a major

Copyright © 2006. Lippincott Williams & Wilkins. *Study Guide to Accompany Essentials of Nursing Research*, by Denise F. Polit and Cheryl Tatano Beck.

research university. A written Explanation of Study Form and an oral explanation were provided to all participants. Participants were informed that completion of the pencil and paper questionnaire packet implied consent to participate in the study. Anonymity of participant responses was ensured. All questionnaires were stored in a locked file cabinet in the investigator's office.

When the data collection site was either a facility or organization, contact people at each location were asked to alert potential participants that the researcher would be coming on a particular day and time. For example, at the McDonald's restaurant, the researcher observed a large group of elder male patrons between the hours of 6:30 AM and 10:30 AM. To begin data collection, the researcher struck up a conversation with one group, explaining the purpose and procedures of the study, and then circulated throughout the restaurant over the ensuing 4-hour period soliciting participation. In contrast, when social groups (i.e., friends and neighbors) known to the investigator were accessed, the men were contacted by telephone, with the investigator ascertaining whether they were interested in participating, and then arrangements were made to meet. On the days of data collection at the senior centers, exercise class, and driving class, the investigator met with each group of potential participants and distributed the explanation of the study form. The form, including the purpose and procedures of the study, was explained. Surveys were self-administered by the participants, with the investigator present to answer questions. Each participant received a token gift of appreciation (a $5.00 restaurant gift certificate).

INSTRUMENTS

The four measures used were compiled into a questionnaire packet in the following order: a 6-item demographics instrument, the 8-item Older Men's Health Program and Screening Inventory (Loeb, 2003), the 44-item Health-Promotion Activities of Older Adults Measure (Padula, 1997a), and the 17-item Health Self-Determinism Index (Cox, 1985). The required reading levels for the instruments ranged from a grade 5.7 to grade 7.9. All were typed in 14-point font with sufficient white space.

DEMOGRAPHICS INSTRUMENT

The demographics instrument, the first instrument in the questionnaire packet, inquired about participants' age, ethnicity/race, marital status, education, income, and the presence of others in the same residence. These demographic variables were chosen for inclusion because prior research (Cox, 1986; Haq & Griffin, 1996) had determined that different combinations of these variables are related significantly to health motivation.

OLDER MEN'S HEALTH PROGRAM AND SCREENING INVENTORY

The Older Men's Health Program and Screening Inventory (Loeb, 2003) inquires about older men's attendance at formal health-promotion programs, participation in age- and

Copyright © 2006. Lippincott Williams & Wilkins. *Study Guide to Accompany Essentials of Nursing Research,* by Denise F. Polit and Cheryl Tatano Beck.

gender-appropriate health screenings, current health conditions, barriers to and anticipated benefits of health-promotion behaviors, and self-ratings of health, healthiness of lifestyle, and satisfaction with current health-promoting behaviors. The first five items are structured as checklists, and participants are to check all responses that apply. The final three questions use 4-point Likert-type scales. One question asks participants to evaluate their health status (poor to excellent). The second question has them rate how healthy their current lifestyle is (never healthy to always healthy), and the third asks them to rate how satisfied they are with their health-promoting behaviors (never satisfied to always satisfied). Reliability testing for these three scaled items yielded a Cronbach alpha of .78 (Loeb, 2003).

HEALTH-PROMOTION ACTIVITIES OF OLDER ADULTS MEASURE

The Health-Promotion Activities of Older Adults Measure (HPAOAM) was chosen for this study because it is designed specifically to measure health-promoting behaviors (lifestyle practices) in older adults. Total scores for the tool are obtained by tallying responses to the 4-point Likert-type items that range from 1 (never) to 4 (always). Possible scores range from 44 to 176, with higher scores indicating greater participation in health-promoting behaviors. Padula (1997a) reported Cronbach's alpha reliability estimates of .87 to .93 for the HPAOAM. In the current investigation, the coefficient alpha was .91.

HEALTH SELF-DETERMINISM INDEX

The Health Self-Determinism Index (HSDI) (Cox, 1985) is a Likert-type survey in which the total score on the instrument is used to measure health motivation. Each item is scored on a scale ranging from 1 (strongly disagree) to 5 (strongly agree). Possible total scores on the HSDI range from 17 to 85, with lower scores indicating more extrinsic motivation and higher scores indicating more intrinsic motivation for health (Cox, 1985). The Cronbach alpha reliability estimates for the HSDI have varied from .82 (Cox, 1985) to .78 (Cox, Miller, & Mull, 1987) to .64 (Loeb et al., 2001) to .61 in the current study.

STATISTICAL ANALYSIS

The Statistical Package for the Social Sciences (SPSS) was used to compute frequency distributions, descriptive statistics, Pearson's product-moment correlations, and stepwise multiple regression analysis. Data were inspected for normalcy. No evidence of multicollinearity was present. Significant differences across data collection sites were found to exist, so a dummy control variable for recruitment site was used in the regression analysis. Because age was significantly different at the rural senior centers, it also was included in the regression equation. The challenge of missing data was addressed by replacing missing values with means for the cases in which variables were scaled in nature. Only one item, anticipated benefits of health-promoting behaviors,

Copyright © 2006. Lippincott Williams & Wilkins. *Study Guide to Accompany Essentials of Nursing Research*, by Denise F. Polit and Cheryl Tatano Beck.

had a concerning amount of missing data (10, 7.5%). Other items in the packet were rarely missed.

■ Results

DESCRIPTION OF PARTICIPANTS

The men ranged in age from 55 to 91 years (mean, 70 years). The majority were White (78.5%), rural (60.7%), and married (66.7%). Levels of education ranged from completion of the fourth grade through completion of doctoral degrees (both MD and PhD), with the most frequently reported level being a high school diploma (21.6%). The participants lived with at least one other person (70.7%) and reported incomes that were "about the same as others my age" (49.3%). Although interval level data on income arguably could have provided more valuable information about the effects of socioeconomic status on health behaviors, categorical data were collected to ensure that participants did not skip the income question.

BIVARIATE ANALYSES

The Pearson product-moment correlation analyses were computed to assess the relations between health motivation and various perceptions regarding health. Total scores on the HSDI were significantly and positively related to self-rated health status ($p \le .001$), self-rated healthiness of lifestyle ($p \le .001$), satisfaction with health-promoting behaviors ($p \le .01$), and total anticipated benefits of health-promoting behaviors ($p \le .05$). After the Bonferroni adjustment for multiple testing (Munro, 1997) was computed, only self-rated health and self-rated healthiness of lifestyle remained significantly correlated with total HSDI scores (Table 1). More intrinsically motivated elderly men assessed their health to be better and their lifestyles to be more healthy.

Through correlation analyses, health motivation was found to have had no significant relation to health-promotion activities, health screening attendance, or health-promotion program attendance. However, health-promotion activities were significantly and positively related to health-promotion program attendance ($p \le .001$) and health screening attendance ($p \le .01$), both withstood the Bonferroni adjustment. Therefore, older men who practiced more health-promotion activities attended significantly more formal health-promotion programs.

Total scores on the HPAOAM were significantly (even with the Bonferroni correction) and positively related to self-rated health status ($p \le .001$), self-rated healthiness of lifestyle ($p \le .001$), satisfaction with health-promoting behaviors ($p \le .001$), and total anticipated benefits from health-promoting behaviors ($p \le .001$). Older men who practiced more health-promotion activities reported better health, more healthy lifestyles, greater satisfaction with their health-promoting behaviors, and more anticipated benefits from health-promoting behaviors. Also, older men who anticipated more benefits from health-promotion behaviors participated in significantly more health screenings ($p \le .01$), a relation that withstood the Bonferroni adjustment.

Copyright © 2006. Lippincott Williams & Wilkins. *Study Guide to Accompany Essentials of Nursing Research*, by Denise F. Polit and Cheryl Tatano Beck.

TABLE 1 Bivariate Correlation Results

Variable		1	2	3	4	5	6	7
1 Health motivation (HSDI)	r	1.00						
	Significant							
2 Health-promoting behaviors (HPAOAM)	r	.130	1.00					
	Significant	.132						
3 Personal evaluation of health (self-rated)	r	.320***[a]	.321****[a]	1.00				
	Significant	.000	.000					
4 Healthiness of lifestyle	r	.325****[a]	.368****[a]	.470****[a]	1.00			
	Significant	.000	.000	.000				
5 Satisfaction with health behaviors	r	.232**	.564****[a]	.470****[a]	.665***[a]	1.00		
	Significant	.007	.000	.000	.000			
6 Total benefits	r	.181*	.485****[a]	.155	.149	.291***[a]	1.00	
	Significant	.043	.000	.085	.098	.001		
7 Total screenings	r	-.064	.265**[a]	-.046	-.069	.008	.272**[a]	1.00
	Significant	.463	.002	.596	.428	.924	.002	
8 Total programs	r	.057	.374****[a]	.005	.049	.170*	.344***[a]	.156
	Significant	.515	.000	.957	.571	.049	.000	.071

Note. HSDI = Health Self-Determinism Index; HPAOAM = Health Promotion Activities of Older Adults Measure.

[a]Those still significant after Bonferroni correction for multiple testing; $p \leq .004$. $n = 135$, except in the correlations with total benefits; there, $n = 124$.

*$p \leq .05$ level (two-tailed). **$p \leq .01$ level (two-tailed). ***$p \leq .001$ level (two-tailed).

Copyright © 2006. Lippincott Williams & Wilkins. *Study Guide to Accompany Essentials of Nursing Research*, by Denise F. Polit and Cheryl Tatano Beck.

TABLE 2 Stepwise Multiple Regression Analysis for Variance in HPAOAM Scores

Step Variable Entered	R^2	F Change	Beta	df_1	df_2
1 Satisfaction	.298	53.153***	.442	1	123
2 Benefits	.414	24.296***	.357	1	122

Note. HPAOAM = Health Promotion Activities of Older Adults Measure; satisfaction = satisfaction with health-promoting behaviors; benefits = total anticipated benefits of health-promoting behaviors.
***$p \leq .001$ level (two-tailed).

MULTIPLE REGRESSION

A stepwise multiple regression analysis was conducted to determine the most predictive equation for health-promotion activities. In addition to the six initially proposed variables, the data collection site variable was compressed into two categories (rural and urban) and entered into the equation, along with age. Only two variables entered the final equation (Table 2). Satisfaction with health-promoting behaviors entered the equation first, explaining 29.8% of the variance. Anticipated benefits of health-promoting behaviors entered second, contributing another 11.6%. Thus, these two variables together explained 41% of the total variance in HPAOAM scores.

Multicollinearity was examined before the stepwise multiple regression analysis. Specifically, the highest correlation coefficient between any two predictor variables was only 0.47. After computation of the step-wise regression, the collinearity tolerances for

TABLE 3 Comparison of White and Nonwhite Older Men

Variable	White, $n = 106$ Mean (SD)	Nonwhite, $n = 29$ Mean (SD)	t	df	p^a
HPAOAM	140.94 (16.91)	145.55 (20.27)	-1.246^b	133	.215
HSDI	53.18 (6.54)	52.34 (7.11)	0.603^b	133	.547
Total benefits	4.49 (2.62)	6.00 (2.24)	-2.813^b	123	.006**d
Income	3.11 (0.98)	2.90 (.77)	-1.104^b	133	.272
Total barriers	0.54 (0.85)	0.97 (1.11)	-1.915^c	133	.063
Total health conditions	3.40 (2.11)	4.97 (2.41)	-3.440^b	133	.001**d
Total screenings	3.83 (1.62)	4.86 (1.51)	-3.078^b	133	.003**d
Total programs	2.44 (2.13)	2.34 (1.82)	0.227^b	133	.820

Note. HSDI = Health Self-Determinism Index; HPAOAM = Health Promotion Activities of Older Adults Measure.
[a]Two-tailed significance.
[b]Equal variance formula.
[c]Unequal variance formula.
[d]Those still significant after Bonferroni correction for multiple testing ($p \leq .006$).
*$p \leq .05$. **$p \leq .01$. ***$p \leq .001$.

Copyright © 2006. Lippincott Williams & Wilkins. *Study Guide to Accompany Essentials of Nursing Research*, by Denise F. Polit and Cheryl Tatano Beck.

TABLE 4 Comparison of White and Nonwhite Older Men

Variable	Rural, $n = 82$ Mean (SD)	Urban, $n = 53$ Mean (SD)	t	df	p^a
HPAOAM	139.39 (16.52)	145.83 (18.89)	-2.100^b	133	.038*
HSDI	53.39 (7.01)	52.41 (6.07)	0.830^b	133	.408
Total benefits	4.19 (2.64)	5.82 (2.23)	-3.597^c	123	$.000^{***d}$
Income	3.11 (1.01)	3.00 (0.83)	0.666^b	133	.507
Total barriers	0.66 (0.92)	0.58 (0.95)	0.449^b	133	.654
Total health conditions	3.44 (2.10)	4.19 (2.44)	-1.897^b	133	.060
Total screenings	3.62 (1.63)	4.72 (1.46)	-3.968^b	133	$.000^{***d}$
Total programs	2.22 (2.13)	2.74 (1.93)	-1.427^b	133	.156

Note. HSDI = Health Self-Determinism Index; HPAOAM = Health Promotion Activities of Older Adults Measure.
[a]Two-tailed significance.
[b]Equal variance formula.
[c]Unequal variance formula.
[d]Those still significant after Bonferroni correction for multiple testing ($p \leq .006$).
$^*p \leq .05.$ $^{**}p \leq .01.$ $^{***}p \leq .001.$

the two-predictor variables were calculated, with a result of 0.916, which indicated a high level of tolerance and thus low collinearity (Munro, 1997).

DIFFERENCES BETWEEN GROUPS

Independent sample *t*-tests were computed to compare Whites with non-Whites (Blacks not of Hispanic origin, Hispanics, Asians/Pacific Islanders, and Native Americans/Alaskan Natives) for differences in mean scores on the major study variables. Three significant differences were noted, and all withstood the Bonferroni adjustment (Table 3). The non-White older men had greater numbers of current health conditions, anticipated more benefits from health-promoting behaviors, and participated in more screening programs. Similarly, rural and urban older men also were assessed for differences in these same variables of interest. Significant differences were found for three of the variables. However, when the Bonferroni value was computed, only two remained statistically significant (Table 4). Urban men were found to anticipate more benefits from health-promoting behaviors and to have participated in a greater number of screenings than their rural counterparts.

■ Discussion

Self-rated health and self-rated healthiness of lifestyle both had significant relations with HSDI scores in this study. The result that healthier men were more intrinsically motivated with regard to their health was consistent with the earlier findings of Haq and Griffin

Copyright © 2006. Lippincott Williams & Wilkins. *Study Guide to Accompany Essentials of Nursing Research*, by Denise F. Polit and Cheryl Tatano Beck.

(1996). The significant and positive relation between HSDI score and self-rated healthiness of lifestyle is particularly noteworthy because the HPAOAM score, which measures a similar construct, was not significantly related to the HSDI score. The finding that men who rate their health as better reported more health-promotion activities is consistent with Padula's (1997b) and Riffle et al.'s (1989) findings of a positive relation between perceived health and health-promoting behaviors.

The absence of a significant relation between health motivation and health-promoting activities is inconsistent with the findings of Haq and Griffin (1996), which showed the two variables as significantly and positively related, and with those of Lucas et al. (2000), who found that lower health motivation scores were significantly related to fewer physical activities in elderly women.

One potential explanation for this discrepancy in findings could be that older men were the population of focus in the current study, whereas the other studies focused solely on either women (Lucas et al., 2000) or elders in general (Haq & Griffin, 1996). These differences support Ratner, Bottorff, Johnson, and Hayduk's (1994) assertion that researchers should not assume men and women have the same motivations for pursuing health-promotion behaviors. A second possible explanation for the discrepancies notes that different instruments were used to measure some of the variables under examination. Lucas et al. (2000) used the HSDI to measure motivation, as in the current study, whereas Haq and Griffin (1996) used the Older Adults Health Motivation instrument, which was unavailable for use upon contact with the authors. In the three prior studies, the Health-Promoting Lifestyle Profile (Walker, Sechrist, & Pender, 1987) was used to measure healthy lifestyle, whereas in the current study, health-promotion activities were operationalized through the HPAOAM (Padula, 1997a). The Health-Promoting Lifestyle Profile was not selected for the current study because in a prior study, elderly participants raised questions as to the appropriateness of some of its items for older adults (Padula, 1997a).

The finding that no significant relation exists between health motivation and health screening participation is inconsistent with the findings from a Fischera and Frank (1994) study, in which health motivation was correlated positively with vigilant mammography screenings. The conflicting findings may be attributed to the fact that the two studies focused on different genders. An alternative explanation is that motivation was measured with the Health Belief Model Scale in the Fischera and Frank (1994) study, whereas the current study operationalized motivation using the HSDI (Cox, 1985). The Health Belief Model Scale was not selected for the current study because the tool measures only general health motivation, thus offering no insights regarding internal or external health motivation.

The lack of a significant correlation between health motivation and health-promotion activities is inconsistent with a study by Loeb et al. (2001), in which those with more intrinsic health motivation were found to attend significantly fewer health-promotion programs. The conflicting results could be attributed to the fact that 69% of the participants in the earlier study were female (Loeb et al., 2001).

Only two predictor variables, satisfaction with health-promoting behaviors and number of anticipated benefits from health-promoting behaviors, were in the final, most predictive equation for HPAOAM scores. The importance of satisfaction with health-promoting behaviors as a predictor for health-promotion activities has not been explored previously.

Copyright © 2006. Lippincott Williams & Wilkins. *Study Guide to Accompany Essentials of Nursing Research*, by Denise F. Polit and Cheryl Tatano Beck.

The finding that older men's anticipation of benefits is in fact predictive of health-promotion activities supports Wieck's (2000) intervention, whereby nurses offer short, intensive education about perceived benefits to encourage more health-promoting behaviors. Similarly, the significant and positive relation found in this study between anticipated benefits and health screening participation supports the exploration of such educational interventions.

Although the non-White participants (primarily African Americans) reported a significantly greater number of current health conditions than their White counterparts, personal evaluations of health did not differ significantly between the two groups. This finding is in agreement with the outcomes of an Armer and Conn (2001) study, which reported that Southern and Midwestern Black and White groups differed significantly in reported numbers of chronic conditions, but that they offered similar self-reports of health, a finding that may be attributed to differing perceptions among cultural groups about normal aging changes. Kaufmann (1996) proposed that older adults tend to define their health by functional abilities, irrespective of diseases present.

The finding that Non-White men participate in significantly more health screenings is noteworthy and conflicts with the Barber, Shaw, Folts, and Taylor (1998) assertion that African American men participate less often in prostate screenings. A relevant anecdotal insight is that many of the African American participants in the current study spontaneously reported that they received their healthcare through the Veterans' Administration. Characteristics of this health system could contribute to their significantly higher rates of screenings.

The discovery that urban and non-White participants anticipated significantly more benefits from health-promoting behaviors and participated in significantly more health screenings may be explained by the fact that the non-Whites were primarily urban dwellers. However, greater screening participation by the urban men, both White and non-White, may be explained by greater service offerings and accessibility in urban centers. These findings support the consideration of multiple interaction effects when rural and urban differences occur and indicate that caution should be exercised in interpreting differences through simplistic urban versus rural generalizations (Morgan, Armstrong, Huppert, Brayne, & Solomou, 2000).

This study has certain limitations. The precision of the older men's responses may have been reduced by inaccurate recall or perceptions of social desirability. Also, the use of a convenience sample limits generalizability. Not all concepts of the Health-Promoting Self-Care System Model were operationalized (i.e., attitudes and social support). Finally, results from reliability testing of the HSDI (Cox, 1985) have been inconsistent.

In conclusion, the findings of this study suggest that promoting self-motivation may be key to increasing older men's perceptions of health and well-being. Further exploration of anticipated benefits as a motivator for health-promotion activities and screening participation is warranted.

This project provides a basis for the development of intervention studies designed to promote: health screening participation, health-promotion program attendance, and health-promoting behavior adoption by older men. Such studies support the *Healthy People 2010* goals of increasing the number of older adults who have participated in one or more organized health-promotion activities during the past year and increasing the years of functional life for older Americans (USDHHS, 2001).

Copyright © 2006. Lippincott Williams & Wilkins. *Study Guide to Accompany Essentials of Nursing Research,* by Denise F. Polit and Cheryl Tatano Beck.

Susan J. Loeb, PhD, RN, is Assistant Professor of Nursing, Department of Nursing, University of Delaware, Newark.

Accepted: January 29, 2004

The author thanks Dr. Sarah Hall Gueldner, Dean and Professor; Decker School of Nursing, Binghamton University—State University of New York (dissertation chairperson); as well as dissertation committee members: Dr. Donald Ford, Professor of Psychology Emeritus and Dean Emeritus, College of Health and Human Development, The Pennsylvania State University; Dr. Judith Hupcey, Assistant Professor of Nursing, The Pennsylvania State University; Dr. Karen Morin, Professor of Nursing, Bronson School of Nursing, Western Michigan University; and Dr. Diana Morris, Associate Professor of Nursing and Associate Director of the University Center on Aging and Health, Frances Payne Bolton School of Nursing, Case Western Reserve University.

Corresponding author: Susan J. Loeb, PhD, RN, Department of Nursing, 367 McDowell Hall, University of Delaware, Newark, DE 19716 (e-mail: sloeb@udel.edu).

REFERENCES

Armer, J. M., & Conn, V. S. (2001). Exploration of spirituality and health among diverse rural elderly individuals. *Journal of Gerontological Nursing, 27*(6), 28–37.

Baker, P. (2001). *Sex and gender matter: From boys to men: The future of men's health*. Conference report. Accessed June 13, 2003 at http://www.medscape.com/viewarticle/415037_2/

Barber, K. R., Shaw, R., Folts, M., & Taylor, K. (1998). Differences between African American and Caucasian men participating in a community-based prostate cancer screening program. *Journal of Community Health, 23*, 441–451.

Bone, P. F. (1991). Identifying mature segments. *The Journal of Services Marketing, 5*(1), 47–60.

Borawski, E. A., Kinney, J. M., & Kahana, E. (1996). The meaning of older adults' health appraisals: Congruence with health status and determinant of mortality. *Journal of Gerontology: Social Sciences, 51B*, S157–S170.

Cohen, J. (1988). *Statistical power analysis for the behavior sciences* (2nd ed.). Hillsdale, NJ: Lawrence Erlbaum Associates.

Cox, C. L. (1982). An interaction model of client health behavior: Theoretical prescription for nursing. *Advances in Nursing Science, 5*(1), 41–56.

Cox, C. L. (1985). The health self-determinism index. *Nursing Research, 34*(3), 177–183.

Cox, C. L. (1986). The interaction model of client health behavior: Application to the study of community-based elders. *Advances in Nursing Science, 9*(1), 40–57.

Cox, C. L., Miller, E. H., & Mull, C. S. (1987). Motivation in health behavior: Measurements, antecedents, and correlates. *Advances in Nursing Science, 9*(4), 1–15.

Diehr, P., Williamson, J., Patrick, D. L., Bild, D. E., & Burke, G. L. (2001). Patterns of self-rated health in older adults before and after sentinel health events. *Journal of the American Geriatrics Society, 49*, 36–44.

Felton, G. M., Parsons, M. A., & Bartoces, M. G. (1997). Demographic factors: Interaction effects on health-promoting behavior and health-related factors. *Public Health Nursing, 14*, 361–367.

Fischera, S. D., & Frank, D. I. (1994). The health belief model as a predictor of mammography screening. *Health Values: Achieving High Level Wellness, 18*(4), 3–9.

Frenn, M. (1996). Older adults' experience of health promotion: A theory for nursing practice. *Public Health Nursing 13*(1), 65–71.

Gabhainn, S. N., Kelleher, C. C., Naughton, A. M., Carter, F., Flanagan, M., & McGrath, M. J. (1999). Sociodemographic variations in perspectives on cardiovascular disease and associated risk factors. *Health Education Research, 14*, 619–628.

Haq, M. B., & Griffin, M. (1996). Health motivation: Key to health-promoting behavior? *The Nurse Practitioner, 21*(11), 155–156.

Copyright © 2006. Lippincott Williams & Wilkins. *Study Guide to Accompany Essentials of Nursing Research*, by Denise F. Polit and Cheryl Tatano Beck.

Idler, E. L., & Kasl, S. V. (1995). Self-ratings of health: Do they also predict change in functional ability? *Journal of Gerontology: Series B: Psychological Sciences & Social Sciences, 50B,* S344–S353.

Kaufmann, J. E. (1996). Personal definitions of health among elderly people: A link to effective health promotion. *Family Community Health, 19*(2), 58–68.

Kosberg, J. I., & Kaye, L. W. (1997). The status of older men: Current perspectives and future projections. In J. I. Kosberg, & L. W. Kaye (Eds.), *Elderly men: Special problems and professional challenges* (pp. 295–307). New York: Springer.

Kosberg, J. I., & Mangum, W. P. (2002). The invisibility of older men in gerontology. *Gerontology and Geriatrics Education, 22*(4), 27–42.

Krout, J. A., McCulloch, B. J., & Kivett, V. R. (1997). Rural older men: A neglected elderly population. In J. I. Kosberg, & L. W. Kaye (Eds.), *Elderly men: Special problems and professional challenges* (pp. 113–130). New York: Springer.

Loeb, S. J. (2003). The older men's health program and screening inventory: A tool for assessing health practices and beliefs. *Geriatric Nursing, 24,* 278–285.

Loeb, S. J., O'Neill, J., & Gueldner, S. H. (2001). Health motivation: A determinant of older adults' attendance at health promotion programs. *Journal of Community Health Nursing, 18,* 151–165.

Loeb, S. J., Penrod, J., Falkenstern, S., Gueldner, S. H., & Poon, L. W. (2003). Supporting older adults living with multiple chronic conditions. *Western Journal of Nursing Research, 25*(1), 8–29.

Lucas, J. A., Orshan, S. A., & Cook, F. (2000). Determinants of health-promoting behavior among women ages 65 and above living in the community. *Scholarly Inquiry for Nursing Practice, 14*(1), 77–109.

Maddox, G. L. (1962). Some correlates of differences in self-assessments of health status among the elderly. *Journal of Gerontology, 17,* 180–185.

Miller, A. M., & Iris, M. (2002). Health promotion attitudes and strategies in older adults. *Health Education and Behavior, 29,* 249–267.

Minkler, M., Schauffler, H., & Clements-Nolle, K. (2000). Health promotion for older Americans in the 21st century. *American Journal of Health Promotion, 14,* 371–379.

Morgan, K., Armstrong, G. K., Huppert, F. A., Brayne, C., & Solomou, W. (2000). Research papers. Healthy ageing in urban and rural Britain: A comparison of exercise and diet. *Age and Ageing, 29,* 341–349.

Munro, B. H. (1997). *Statistical methods for health care research* (3rd ed.). Philadelphia: Lippincott.

Orem, D. E. (1985). *Nursing: Concepts of practice* (3rd ed.). New York: McGraw-Hill.

Padula, C. A. (1997a). Development of the health promotion activities of older adults measure. *Public Health Nursing, 14*(2), 123–128.

Padula, C. A. (1997b). Predictors of participation in health promotion activities by elderly couples. *Journal of Family Nursing, 3*(1), 88–106.

Pender, N. J. (1987). *Health promotion in nursing practice* (2nd ed.). Norwalk, CT: Appleton & Lange.

Ratner, P. A., Bottorff, J. L., Johnson, J. L., & Hayduk, L. A. (1994). The interaction effects of gender within the Health Promotion Model. *Research in Nursing and Health, 17,* 341–350.

Riffle, K. L., Yoho, J., & Sams, J. (1989). Health-promoting behaviors, perceived social support, and self-reported health of Appalachian elderly. *Public Health Nursing, 6*(4), 204–211.

Rosenstock, I. M. (1960). What research in motivation suggests for public health. *American Journal of Public Health, 50,* 295–302.

Simmons, S. J. (1990). The Health-Promoting Self-Care System Model: Directions for nursing research and practice. *Journal of Advanced Nursing 15,* 1162–1166.

U. S. Census Bureau. (2000). Race and Hispanic or Latino. Geographic area: Pennsylvania: Urban/rural and inside/outside metropolitan area. Accessed September 7, 2003 at http://factfinder.census.gov/servlet/GCTTable?_ts = 81015591484.

U. S. Department of Health and Human Services. (2001). *Healthy People 2010.* Boston: Jones and Bartlett.

Walker, S. N., Sechrist, K. R., & Pender, N. J. (1987). The health-promoting lifestyle profile: Development and psychometric characteristics. *Nursing Research, 36*(2), 76–81.

Copyright © 2006. Lippincott Williams & Wilkins. *Study Guide to Accompany Essentials of Nursing Research,* by Denise F. Polit and Cheryl Tatano Beck.

Watson, N., & Pulliam, L. (2000). Transgenerational health promotion. *Holistic Nursing Practice, 14*(4), 1–11.

Wieck, K. L. (2000). Health promotion for inner-city minority elders. *Journal of Community Health Nursing, 17*(3), 131–139.

Wrobel, A. J., & Shapiro, N. E. K. (1999). Conducting research with urban elders: Issues of recruitment, data collection, and home visits. *Alzheimer Disease and Associated Disorders, 13*(Suppl 1), S34–S38.

Zabalegui, A. (1994). Aging matters: Barriers to health. *Nursing Times, 90*(1), 58–61.

Copyright © 2006. Lippincott Williams & Wilkins. *Study Guide to Accompany Essentials of Nursing Research,* by Denise F. Polit and Cheryl Tatano Beck.

"THE PEOPLE KNOW WHAT THEY WANT"

An Empowerment Process of Sustainable, Ecological Community Health

Katherine N. Bent, RN, PhD, CNS

Community-focused nurses routinely confront issues of environmental hazards in the context of the community. Limits to disciplinary knowledge about health, environment, and community constrain practice for many who are interested in ways to promote community health across a spectrum of diverse needs and contexts, including the context of the environment. The purpose of the reported critical ethnography was to explore the relationships among health, environment, and culture from the cultural context of one community. Findings highlight the emancipatory, yet ambiguous, process through which this community transformed individual symptoms of illness into an experience and examination of community environment and community health. The significance of this work lies in inductively building knowledge and theory about these relationships and community empowerment for community-focused nursing.

■ **Key words:** *community health, critical theory, empowerment, environmental health, ethnography*

Never doubt that a small group of thoughtful committed citizens can change the world; indeed, it is the only thing that ever has.

Margaret Mead

Community-focused nurses routinely confront issues of environmental health in the context of the community. An important element of practicing in this context is knowing how and being able to address community-level issues to improve individual and community health and health experiences. Limits to disciplinary knowledge about health, environment, and even community constrain practice for many who are interested in ways to

Reprinted with permission from *Advances in Nursing Science* 2003; 26 [3]: 215–226.

Copyright © 2006. Lippincott Williams & Wilkins. *Study Guide to Accompany Essentials of Nursing Research*, by Denise F. Polit and Cheryl Tatano Beck.

promote health across a spectrum of diverse needs and contexts, including the context of the environment. The purpose of the reported ethnographic study was to explore the relationships among health, environment, culture, and health policy from the cultural context of one community. The significance of this work lies in building knowledge and theory about these relationships for community-focused nursing. Findings of this study address community responses to environmental health hazards as well as the quality and safety of the physical environment from the perspective of how communities interact with the environment in their cultural patterns of living.

▪ Background

CONCEPTUAL FRAMEWORK

The current study was developed from a perspective of human science, a tradition in which knowledge is understood to be truthful within a particular context. The following concepts were expected to be important to the context of the study and were reviewed for background understanding: culture, community health, and environment.

Culture

Culture is a broad anthropological and social concept that generally refers to the dynamic, but tenacious over time, social context of beliefs, values, ways of knowing, and patterns of behavior characteristic of a designated population group.[1,2] The interpretive significance of understanding culture lies not in seeking a static, causal predictor of individual or group behavior, but rather in understanding the meaning of living in the culture and exploring the conditions by which cultural values, norms, and truths are constructed.[3,4]

Community Health

Although community is part of our life experience, the idea of community remains elusive and can mean many things, particularly in a health care context.[5-8] Monroe additionally noted that in a politically charged environment, claims of community often become moral claims that may divide people more than it brings them together.[6] This effect has serious consequences for questions of public health, for the basis for health lies in communities where environmental resources are available and where a sense of cohesion can bring about distribution of these resources to achieve sustainable health.[9-11]

Although nursing models have primarily understood human health experiences to be individual rather than communitarian in nature, there is a perspective of health that includes community dimensions and contexts and looks to understand determinants of health in order to apply the concepts of health and caring to a community.[12-14] From this perspective, health is a dynamic experience that includes personal, social, political, environmental, and cultural factors, as well as persons' and communities' responses and interactions with these factors.

Community health nurses have a tradition of actively creating and strengthening partnerships for health promotion and community health.

Copyright © 2006. Lippincott Williams & Wilkins. *Study Guide to Accompany Essentials of Nursing Research*, by Denise F. Polit and Cheryl Tatano Beck.

Community health experiences are complex and dynamic experiences that need to be understood in the broad environmental, sociocultural, and political contexts in which they develop. Nursing research is needed to explore community health experiences and relationships in these contexts, to address multi- and interdisciplinary efforts toward partnership and community development, as well as to describe what dimensions of community are relevant to their involvement in health development.[15]

Environment

Environment is one of the primary determinants of health, yet scientific understanding of the potential adverse health effects of environmental hazards is incomplete.[16] In the theoretical and conceptual frameworks of nursing, environment includes the natural environment and social, economic, cultural, and political structures that are the landscape and geography of human experience.[17] Nurses are increasingly expected to be informational and political resources for individuals and community organizations that are becoming active to protect local environmental health experiences.[16] Few researchers, nurse or nonnurse, have published data and findings that support environmental health in the clinical practice of nursing, and the literature as it exists is fragmented and isolated.[16]

SETTING

This critical ethnographic study was conducted in the San José community, an urban *barrio* (a Spanish-speaking neighborhood in a city or town in the United States especially in the Southwest) located on the Rio Grande River in Albuquerque, NM. This community is of interest because of strong, ongoing relationships between this predominantly Hispanic (89.7%),[18] low-income community and the New Mexico Department of Health to develop and implement community-based environmental health programs and community-focused health and development strategies.

The community is geographically marked by the AT&SF railroad, one interstate highway, and the Rio Grande River. San José is zoned to support both residential and industrial use. The industry here facilitates high levels of sustained growth throughout Albuquerque and includes oil refineries, tanneries, manufacturing, and salvage yards. Because of a heavy concentration of toxic waste sites, 2 locales in San José were listed on the Superfund National Priorities list in the late 1980s and 1990s. This was both practically and symbolically tragic to a community that was first developed and long defined by agriculture. The concentration of environmental pollutants and industrial contamination in San José caused land use to decline and property values to drop. The once prosperous agricultural community of San José was zoned as a federal Pocket of Poverty neighborhood where the community environment is now polluted not only by industrial emissions and toxic chemicals, but also by drug deals, gang activity, prostitution, and high crime rates. In this community, environmental, social, economic, cultural, and political conditions and changes are interconnected as the total community environment has become increasingly hazardous. The Albuquerque San José Community Awareness Council, Inc (ASJCAC or Awareness Council), is a grassroots organization, formed in 1988 in response to environmental health hazards in the community and concerns over Superfund site status. Years of grassroots organizing, however, have brought dramatic

Copyright © 2006. Lippincott Williams & Wilkins. *Study Guide to Accompany Essentials of Nursing Research*, by Denise F. Polit and Cheryl Tatano Beck.

changes in remediating hazardous industrial sites, crime rates, abandoned or derelict properties, public services, and other improvements in quality of life for people who live there.

As a study site, San José was selected because this urban, culturally and ethnically diverse community addresses a key assumption of the Healthy Cities movement, that is, when people have the opportunity to work out their own locally defined health problems, they will find sustainable solutions.[19] As an example of grassroots political action, a study of change in San José may elicit how actions related to health might work in other communities. The study was guided by the following research question: what is the experience in San José such that community health initiatives generated through local environmental, health, and development concerns have been sustained over time?

■ Research Design

In this study, ethnographic design and methods were used to access the depth of cultural experience as well as both locally and externally interpreted meanings of social, economic, and political phenomena. The study and procedures for obtaining informed consent were reviewed and approved by the Colorado Multiple Institutional Review Board (COMIRB). The investigator conducted all aspects of the research herself, as described in the following discussion.

DATA GENERATION

Data were generated in monthly field trips of 3 to 10 days over a period of 10 months, between 1999 and 2000. Data generation opportunities followed ethnographic methodology and included interviews, participant observation, field notes, examination of artifacts and existing documents, and photographic images of the community.[20–23] Following the suggestion of Austin, I also solicited maps of San Jose drawn or filled in by interview participants.[22] The maps were used to visualize some micro and macro aspects of the community, including perceived boundaries of the community, places participants perceive to be "problems" in the community, places participants go every day or almost every day, and places participants believe are important to the culture or history of the community.

Sample

A sample of 33 primary participants was purposively selected for this study. Initial key informants included 5 employees and board members of the ASJCAC, elected officials, and government advisors to the Awareness Council. Following interviews with these key informants, sampling continued with others they had recommended for inclusion in the study and with theoretical decisions made from ongoing data analysis. The final sample of 33 included 19 women; 30 participants were self-identified "Hispanics" and 3 were self-identified "Anglos" who lived, had family of origin, attended religious services and community functions, or worked in San José over an extended period of time. The

Copyright © 2006. Lippincott Williams & Wilkins. *Study Guide to Accompany Essentials of Nursing Research*, by Denise F. Polit and Cheryl Tatano Beck.

majority self-identified as Catholic and many had attended high school for some period, although few had graduated and some had no formal education. Participants ranged in age from 23 to 82 years of age and those who had lived in the community had often been in the same house for 15 to 37 years. Ten additional secondary participants included individuals who worked with residents of San José or had time-limited or single issue exposure to the activities and concerns of the community, for example, media or industrial neighbors.

Methods

Each primary participant was interviewed from 1 to 4 times for approximately 1 hour each time. These interviews were generally audiotaped, although several were recorded only in field notes. Lead questions in early interviews were broad and asked participants to reflect on questions like "What's it like to live in San José?" or "Is San José a healthy place to live?" for example. As the interviews and the study progressed, questions evolved to inquire about if and how participants thought issues of growth were related to health in San José or how people in San José communicated around local problems or issues. Interviews were transcribed and identifying information was removed; transcripts, field notes, and any external, text-based documents were entered into the NUD*IST© software program for subsequent coding and analysis.

Participant observation included attendance at Mass and other church services, public meetings, Awareness Council meetings, neighborhood fairs or celebrations, as well as daily life in the community. Field notes recorded during participant observation activities were used to aid interpretation as well as uncover bias. Historical and contemporary artifacts were obtained from a variety of sources and examined. Items included newsletters from the Awareness Council, pertinent legislation, contracts between the Awareness Council and the health department or between the Awareness Council and their subcontractors, Environmental Protection Agency publications, community planning documents, library and museum collections, works from local authors, and media coverage.

Photographs were used both in interviewing and analysis. For example, most participants in this study were very long-term residents of the community, and some shared family photographs that parenthetically illustrated changes in the community over time. These photos would then often prompt participants' own reflections on the nature or experience of changes in the community and the environment. Researcher photos were also used in analysis to enhance participants' descriptions of their community or to make stated values or experiences visible. In analysis new images were viewed alongside old or photos were analyzed for "natural," "constructed," or "empty" environmental space within specific images. Participants who were photographed gave additional consent and were given the opportunity to specify acceptable uses for the photographs.

DATA ANALYSIS

Data analysis was initiated with data generation and continued throughout the study. Analytic activities began with reflecting, reading and re-reading the data, and organizing the data into categories using codes. Categories were created for events, processes, characteristics, quotes, emotions, and responses, for example, using both participants' words

Copyright © 2006. Lippincott Williams & Wilkins. *Study Guide to Accompany Essentials of Nursing Research*, by Denise F. Polit and Cheryl Tatano Beck.

and researcher typologies.[24] A segment of text would generally contain several coded categories. Categories were analyzed for central ideas. When categories grouped around similar ideas, domains, or locally specific, cultural symbols of shared meaning emerged. Following identification and analysis of cultural domains, the data were analyzed for cultural themes. Themes are broader units of thought that describe experience from within the cultural context, and unify contributing domains and experiences.[25] Strategies used to inductively generate domains and themes included narrative analysis, relational analysis, examination of metaphors, and content analysis.

Trustworthiness[26] of the findings is enhanced by prolonged engagement, multiple interviews with several participants, deliberate inclusion of points of view from individuals known to disagree with ideas held by the Awareness Council and other primary participant organizations, member checks of ongoing analysis, and peer debriefing with senior researchers familiar with the ethnographic design or phenomena of interest.

■ Findings

From ethnographic analysis, 5 cultural domains, 4 cultural themes, and 1 integrative theme about community experiences of health, environment, culture, and health policy emerged. The focus of this article is selected thematic findings of this study, with particular emphasis on the integrative theme. Discovery of themes involved a process of critical reflection on the domains as well as a return to the stories told by the participants to elicit what has been called a *thick* description.[27] Cultural themes reconstruct aspects of community health and quality of life in San José; the identification of an overarching integrative theme recontextualized these findings within the holistic experiences of the community.

INTEGRATIVE THEME: IN SAN JOSÉ, SUSTAINABLE COMMUNITY HEALTH EMBODIES AND REFLECTS AN EMPOWERMENT PROCESS

The integrative theme takes shape because that there is a story of community struggle to be told. Although the people of San José all live this story and the shared experiences that fill the outlines of the story, there was no single participant who filled the role of community historian. This is a story of community self-efficacy, of pride and self-reliance, and of people struggling together in different ways to solve many kinds of community problems.

Although the history of the community's experience reaches to the early 1800s, the current experience begins in 1983 when the South Valley Superfund Site was identified as New Mexico's first Superfund site after routine water sampling by the City of Albuquerque found 2 contaminated supply wells. In 1987, the Environmental Protection Agency installed a municipal supply well; however, individuals who lived and worked in San José continued to experience symptoms such as stomach upsets, repiratory difficulties, or skin rashes and were starting to wonder about the relationship of symptoms to the hazards in the environment. Additionally, persons living in the community noticed that the water in their homes was foul smelling and foul tasting and that frequently the

Copyright © 2006. Lippincott Williams & Wilkins. *Study Guide to Accompany Essentials of Nursing Research,* by Denise F. Polit and Cheryl Tatano Beck.

air also had an offensive odor. These individual experiences were shared with significant others and talked about in families. Individuals with health concerns may have seen health care providers for specific complaints, but interactions with primary care providers and local public health practitioners were episodic.

The concerns voiced about foul water particularly caught the attention of one parish priest who forged formal ties with environmental special interest groups in the city. Members of this new partnership solicited participation from a few committed community members, but could not achieve a broad base of community support, in part because community members felt these outsiders were condescending and disrespectful of local knowledge. In the words of one participant, "The job he [the priest] was doing, it was for the benefit of the community, but he wasn't going about it the right way." When initial organizing efforts were rewarded with funding from the Environmental Protection Agency and the state of New Mexico, the ASJCAC was created, and community members became increasingly interested, active, and critical of previously accepted processes.

Funding at last brought the experiences and issues of the people in San José to the consciousness of state public health officials who were the administrative funnel for some of the funds. In developing the contractual scope of work for these monies, officials saw themselves as facilitating the goals of the Awareness Council but also bringing their proposed projects "more in line with the Departmental mission," which was "more about health promotion than environmental health issues." The priest's parish appointment ended and community members who were volunteering time, effort, and local knowledge encouraged one of their own to apply for the Executive Director position of the Awareness Council. With this step, control visibly started to shift to the community.

Under new, community-based leadership and with the Department of Health advocating for and supporting a wide range of health promotion activities, the focus of the Awareness Council evolved. Through focused contracts with environmental experts, the Awareness Council continues as a community "watchdog" for the technical issues and advocacy concerns regarding Superfund activities in the community. Beyond Superfund activities, however, the Awareness Council now has an agenda that includes other issues that affect the community environment: community policing, court monitoring, speed humps next to the elementary school, paving dirt roads, traffic lights on busy roads, fair property tax assessments, police and fire substations in the community, voter registration, housing services, employment opportunities, cultural promotion and awareness, letters to absentee landlords with problem tenants, and closing a notorious bar. It includes all of these issues precisely because, in the words of one participant, "*la gente sabe [lo] que quiere* [the people know what they want]." Through these kinds of activities, the practical meaning of the word environment is expressed as inclusive of soil and water contamination, but also more contextually specific to the experiences of San José. Community members themselves take these efforts very seriously: "this is a real community, with real problems that can be provided real solutions, I guess is what I'm saying. And that's why our work is very important." These efforts rely on and are reinforced by appraisals of successful outcomes by both the community itself and outside organizations.

The Awareness Council letterhead proclaims that the work of the Awareness Council is "to empower our community to solve our own problems." This is, in fact, a radical departure from the traditional structure of power and politics in San José in which one powerful individual controlled all aspects of community functioning. While the Awareness

Copyright © 2006. Lippincott Williams & Wilkins. *Study Guide to Accompany Essentials of Nursing Research,* by Denise F. Polit and Cheryl Tatano Beck.

Council has been the largest, best funded, and most visible example of community activism and empowerment, it is by no means the only one in San José. The actual link to empowerment lies in the community reclaiming the sense of accomplishment from doing the work to change. And the only way to achieve that sense of accomplishment is to do the work. As one woman with a long history of volunteering in the community said:

> We are proud, but sometimes we get lazy and we don't speak up. We think somebody else is going to do it for us. And we have to do it ourselves, we have to get out there and talk and voice what we feel, what needs to be done. And sometimes we worry about how we will sound, but if it's coming from the heart, then that does make a difference. If you truly believe it.

One particular achievement illustrates this community power and empowerment. In the fall of 1998, the Executive Director of the Awareness Council, who is a long-time resident of San José, won an at-large elected position on the city-wide School Board, despite a large field of candidates, and without benefit of any media endorsements. As one government observer noted:

> All power is perceived. I've always said that, because I see people that they've pointed to and say 'oh, he or she is so powerful.' And they couldn't get you one vote, you know? But it's just the perception. And then you have some people here that it's not a perception. I mean, it's really there. And proof of the pudding is, you have somebody run from San José, and win you know. I thought it was tremendous.

That a woman, of color, from one of the city's poorest neighborhoods won this election makes a powerful statement about this community's commitment and their ability to act as a community on that commitment to achieve positive outcome that is likely to change their experiences and their world.

As the emphasis in community activities continues to evolve from solving crises to maintaining successful intervention programs and proactively addressing future community needs, not only is the environment itself seen more broadly by community members, but these environmental issues are understood to be issues of community quality of life that are worth pursuing. New community development initiatives continue to become possible, for example, applying for federal Brownfields funding to address redevelopment in areas that are or are perceived to be contaminated. While milestones such as the Board of Education election signal levels of success, funding continues from both Environmental Protection Agency and the state to support these activities.

SUPPORTING THEMES

There Is a Persistent Sense of Community in San José

People in the community hold an abiding sense about the "essence" of San José, in which the community is grounded in the people and the culture. One way this sense of community takes form is through historical connection to place. As one participant observed, "this is a good place, this is a real place, this is where Albuquerque started."

Copyright © 2006. Lippincott Williams & Wilkins. *Study Guide to Accompany Essentials of Nursing Research*, by Denise F. Polit and Cheryl Tatano Beck.

Alternatively, it may be: "peoples' memories—that's what the foundation of San José is. Both the good and the bad." Because this sense of community seems to render the more recent presence of Mexican immigrants invisible, it is somewhat idealized and exclusionary, particularly in light of increasing tension and changing cultural, community dynamics. However, members of the community perceive this abiding community identity to be a strength of their community.

There Is an Uncertain Sense of the Future in San José

Along with having a strong sense of community, participants reflected both optimism and wariness, culminating in an uncertain sense of what the future holds for San José. Uncertainty is expressed in 2 ways: the first is related to the place and its structures and systems, and the second is focused on the people and organizational relations within the community. One city bureaucrat observed:

> The city's providing these incentives for businesses to come, but I guess the argument comes back to what kind of jobs that it provided. They're providing $5.00 an hour jobs to get tax breaks or are they going to be providing $10 an hour jobs where a family could live on it.

Although San José has been marked by self-reinforcing problems of poverty and stigma, the culture and the tradition of the people who live there again come to be understood as a source of strength to shape the future positively. As one participant noted,

> I think the assets of San José have been downplayed to some degree, but because of the history of San José, that's where I think the potential is the strongest. Because with the history comes a lot of integrity and people who feel very, very strongly about San José.

Participants wondered whether the community will be able to use these assets and strengths effectively, for although the community is committed to self-determination, there are divisive fractures among community populations. One participant cited Mexican immigrants as an example:

> Well, see, with the migration of so many Mexican nationals into the neighborhood, I think if they are here on an illegal status, I think they'll mistrust anybody, so that's why a lot of them keep in the background. I think what's wrong with these people is they're scared to come out . . . in this area there's a lot of prejudice.

Even though this resident sees 2 sides to a perceived problem, it is interesting to note the inferred progression: the future rests on participation from community members; Mexicans, for whatever reason, aren't participating; therefore they are the problem.

Community Health Is a Multidimensional Experience That Can Be Described as Quality of Life from the Perspective of People Who Live There

Quality of life has traditionally been understood as an individual perception; however, participants were vocal about the existence of a community quality of life. They were

Copyright © 2006. Lippincott Williams & Wilkins. *Study Guide to Accompany Essentials of Nursing Research*, by Denise F. Polit and Cheryl Tatano Beck.

articulate in positioning community quality of life within a multidimensional perspective. Participants in this study identify quality of life in San José not only by opposing it to qualities or experiences perceived as negative, but also through the presence of or potential for positive qualities in the community, as described by this resident:

> What makes up a healthy community? A healthy community is where everybody gets along [pause]. No, a healthy community is where children are feeling good about going outside. They have bicycles; they play in their yard; they can go across the street to their neighbors' houses and play; they're getting good educations. That we have good jobs and livable wages. We don't want to make this into another part of the city; we want to make sure that we continue like San José, but safe. We don't want exposed wires. If they want a GED class, in Spanish, swimming lessons, whatever. And it might seem so minute, but it's a part of it. All of it.

People who live in the community express a perspective of community health as inclusive of many dimensions of daily life, including crime, socioeconomic opportunity, education, toxins in the environment, local infrastructure, and the culture of the community itself. Community-focused attention to the diverse quality of life needs is deliberate and goal-directed on the part of community members and organizations.

SUMMARY OF THEMES

These themes paint a picture of life in a community with both a strong history and tradition and an uncertain future. The community has successfully used cultural and other internal strengths to sustain health and quality of life initiatives throughout periods of change and challenge. The community has also used its strength to redefine local experiences of community health and of the community environment into a central experience of quality of life. The integrative theme, "In San José, sustainable community health embodies and reflects an empowerment process," represents these themes and the importance of the Awareness Council in shaping community life and health. The development and change reflected in community experience in San José support an empowerment process in which the growth of the community is linked to growth of individuals who participate in community process. The story of community empowerment is a synthesis drawn from this dynamic dialectic between the individuals and the collective.

■ Discussion

SOCIAL CAPITAL

Putnam attributes a significant portion of community well being to the presence of social capital, which is a series of networks and community norms that enable community members to work together effectively to achieve common goals, such as improved community health and quality of life.[28] There are 2 types of social capital: bonding capital and bridging capital.[28] Bonding capital strengthens relationships among people or

Copyright © 2006. Lippincott Williams & Wilkins. *Study Guide to Accompany Essentials of Nursing Research*, by Denise F. Polit and Cheryl Tatano Beck.

groups who already know each other; this has also been called the sociocultural milieu of a community.[29] Bridging capital brings together people or groups who do not know each other, and has been linked to institutional infrastructure.[29] Putnam's theory of social capital is that the more people connect with each other, the more they will trust each other and the better off they will be, both collectively and individually.[28] In this sense, success reinforces cooperation and trust, although at a risk of excluding some in the community. Results from the current study substantiate this concept of social capital in San José as well as suggest that members of the community are aware of the practical value of being defined as a community with social capital. Relying solely on social capital to explain success, however, also implies that a lack of social capital is responsible for lower levels of success seen in some initiatives. Such an implication would serve to further condemn the community for generations of sociopolitical and environmental injustice. Such reliance also negates subtle but important findings that suggest the sense of community may be idealized and therefore as exclusive as it is inclusive.

EMPOWERMENT

Empowerment has become part of modern lexicon and jargon, but it means many things to many people in different contexts. Within the discourse of empowerment, there are levels of community participation that range from passive compliance through tokenism to a true sharing of decisionmaking.[30] Freire introduced a dialectical understanding of empowerment as encompassing both individual and social dimensions.[31] Israel and colleagues[32] have developed and tested a measure of community empowerment through a scale of perceived control. By measuring perceived control in one urban community, they concluded that action at the community level results in enhanced collective problem-solving capabilities and increased influence and control over resources.

The current study provided an assessment of the richness and complexity of community empowerment that could not have been captured by scales or instruments. In addition, this study addresses culturally specific ideas of both community empowerment and community health that may be inaccessible through simple aggregating of individual responses on standardized measures. In San José, empowerment is an interactive, social process of change in which the community is transformed as people who participate are transformed. Empowerment, then, is not static, nor is it a panacea intervention to be inflicted upon others to solve community problems, but rather empowerment is an invitation to think differently about how to solve problems that endanger health in many ways. These findings suggest concurrence between lay and professional understanding of the concept of empowerment.

Community empowerment is not an alternative to understanding and taking action at higher levels. Observations of community experiences in San José illuminate larger problems posed by environmental and other injustices; for example, if residents of San José are empowered to rid their community of toxic waste, the environment of another community suffers from the "downstream" effects of receiving it. Nor is community empowerment a justification for reducing institutionalized services and support. To place responsibility solely with the community assumes the community alone is willing, able, and morally obligated to take responsibility for all community health experiences. These questions of emphasis remain relevant as national policies "decentralize," state policies

Copyright © 2006. Lippincott Williams & Wilkins. *Study Guide to Accompany Essentials of Nursing Research*, by Denise F. Polit and Cheryl Tatano Beck.

"localize," and individuals and communities are told they hold more responsibility than ever for their own health experiences, thus also implying that the individual or single community is responsible for the success or failure of public health policy. Community health is ecological and requires social, physical, political, cultural, environmental, spiritual, and economic supports that reflect the context in which community health problems developed. In this sense, empowerment must focus on strengthening the skills people need to regain power in their lives.

The National Civic League has defined *capacity* as including the processes, products, and abilities that enable those entities that contribute to the production of community health to perform varied functions.[33] This concept refers to the capacity of a community as a whole and includes people, system, and infrastructure. Although this definition of community capacity explicitly focuses on health, it also treats health as a commodity rather than as an experience of the community. Findings from the current study on the meaning and pride communities attach to community health, quality of life, and empowerment processes and experiences complement the National Civic League definition of capacity and may also assist other communities in envisioning, understanding, or developing their own definitions of this abstract concept of capacity.

LIMITATIONS OF THE STUDY

This study offers insight into the processes of community health and quality of life in the cultural context of one community. It has been noted, however, that an apparent ecological or structural effect may in fact arise from individual-level processes rather than those at the level of the community as a whole. Additionally, because this study focused attention on a single community, applicability of these findings to other communities must be undertaken with careful consideration. Finally, my position as an Anglo researcher and outsider to the community may offer a limitation to the study. Although inquiry was undertaken over a period of time, and despite the enthusiasm and pride with which participants told their stories, it is possible that there are community members who would not participate or others who withheld information because of my status.

IMPLICATIONS FOR NURSING

Community health is complex, multidimensional, and cannot be addressed in isolation. Nurses would do well to include and address within theory, practice, and research the broad range of factors and dimensions of environment, health, and well-being that communities themselves identify as defining the health of the community. It is these very experiences that are also likely to differ from the phenomena and perspectives that other professional public health disciplines address.

A model developed inductively from the current study helps not only address the question of sustained success that drove this study, but also illustrates the empowerment process by which individual experiences (symptoms of illness and disease) were transformed into an examination and experience of community environment and community health (Fig 1). In this model, individual and community experiences are linked and contribute to the perception of risk, including for some, the perception of those structural

Copyright © 2006. Lippincott Williams & Wilkins. *Study Guide to Accompany Essentials of Nursing Research,* by Denise F. Polit and Cheryl Tatano Beck.

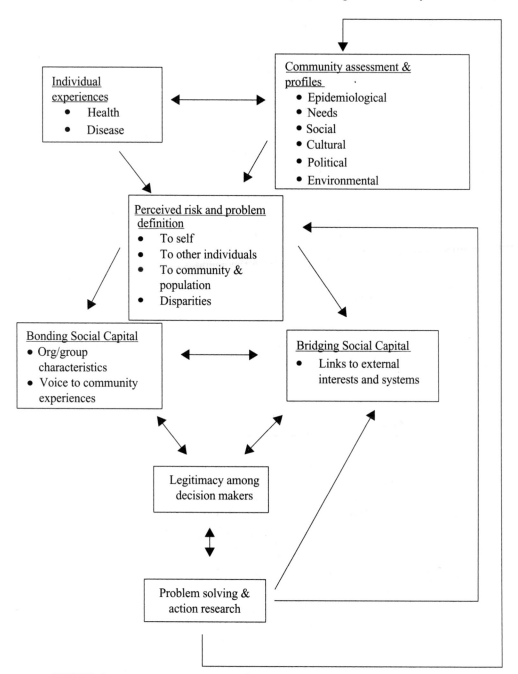

FIGURE 1. An empowerment process of sustainable, ecological community health.

Copyright © 2006. Lippincott Williams & Wilkins. *Study Guide to Accompany Essentials of Nursing Research*, by Denise F. Polit and Cheryl Tatano Beck.

factors and processes that enhance inequality and vulnerability to risk. When elements of risk are perceived to self, others, and community, it prompts actions that create social capital. Social capital provides and reinforces legitimacy in various policy arenas, and legitimacy in turn facilitates problem solving. Problem solving offers important feedback for redefining community experiences and risk perception, while further supporting the opportunity presented by social capital.

This model offers a way to look critically at both community problems and sustainable solutions and offers several points at which nurses can be influential in promoting community-based and community-focused health. First, community health nurses are skilled in conducting and disseminating community assessment, which is an integral part of helping individuals see the importance of their own experience as it contributes to a larger community context. Second, by defining risk, inequality, and vulnerability in communities, nurses have an opportunity to add knowledge of injustice and disparate experiences of health and environment among racial, ethnic, gender, or other minority groups. Third, nurses can assist as communities build bridging social capital by helping them express their concerns in ways that fall within the agendas of health care, governmental, and other policy systems. Fourth, by giving voice to community-based and community-focused dimensions of health and environment that may not find expression or legitimacy elsewhere, nurses can contribute to the bonding social capital that draws and keeps individuals together in a shared community health experience. And finally, at the point of problem solving, nurses who engage in action research can help communities and relevant agencies identify policy and strategies likely to be meaningful to all stakeholders, successful and just.

▪ Conclusion

Findings and theoretical analysis from the reported study reflect the local history of this community and highlight the emancipatory, yet ambiguous, process through which this community transformed individual symptoms of illness into an experience and examination of community environment and community health. Through an empowerment process in which the individuals and the community struggle and grow stronger together, the people of San José have given voice, structure, and action to their concerns. Their success may serve as a model for other communities seeking to define and address a wide variety of health concerns and as a focal point for community-focused nursing theory, practice, and research.

From the VA Eastern Colorado Health Care System, and the University of Colorado Health Sciences Center School of Nursing, Denver, Colo.
This research was supported by a grant from the National Institute of Nursing Research, 5F31NR007269–03.
Special thanks to the residents of the San José who continue to work for sustainable, ecological community health and to J. Kathy Magilvy, RN, PhD, FAAN, for critique of an earlier version of this manuscript.
Corresponding author: Katherine N. Bent, RN, PhD, CNS, VAECHCS, MS 118, 1055 Clemont St, Denver, CO 80220 (e-mail: Katherine.bent@med.va.gov).

Copyright © 2006. Lippincott Williams & Wilkins. *Study Guide to Accompany Essentials of Nursing Research*, by Denise F. Polit and Cheryl Tatano Beck.

REFERENCES

1. Kleinman A. *Patients and Healers in the Context of Culture.* Berkeley: University of California Press; 1980.
2. Leininger MM. *Culture Care Diversity and Universality Theory: A Theory of Nursing.* New York: National League for Nursing; 1983.
3. Geertz C. *The Interpretation of Cultures.* New York: Basic Books; 1973.
4. Thomas J. *Doing Critical Ethnography.* Newbury Park, Calif: Sage; 1993.
5. Sheilds LE, Lindsey AE. Community health promotion nursing practice. *Adv Nurs Sci.* 1998;20:23–36.
6. Monroe JA. Enemies of the people: the moral dimension to public health. *J Health Polit Policy Law.* 1997;22:993–1020.
7. Kirkpatrick FG. *Community: A Trinity of Models.* Washington, DC: Georgetown University Press; 1986.
8. Peterson MA. Community meaning and opportunity, and learning for the future. *J Health Polit Policy Law.* 1997;22:933–936.
9. Milio N. Developing nursing leadership in health policy. *J Prof Nurs.* 1989;5:315–321.
10. World Health Organization. *Report of the International Conference on Primary Health Care.* Geneva: WHO; 1978.
11. Citrin T. Public health—community or commodity? Reflections on healthy communities. *Am J Public Health.* 1998;88:351–352.
12. Craig C. Community determinants of health for rural elderly. *Public Health Nurs.* 1994;12:366–373.
13. Pender NJ. *Health Promotion in Nursing Practice.* 3rd ed. Stamford, Conn: Appleton & Lang; 1996.
14. Salmon ME. Public health policy: creating a healthy future for the American public. *Fam Community Health.* 1995;8:1–11.
15. Oakley P. *Community Involvement in Health Development: An Examination of the Critical Issues.* Geneva: World Health Organization; 1989.
16. Institute of Medicine. In: Pope M, Snyder MA, Mood LH, eds., *Nursing, Health, and the Environment.* Washington, DC: National Academy Press; 1995.
17. Chopoorian TJ. Reconceptualizing the environment. In Moccia P, ed. *New Approaches to Theory Development.* New York: National League for Nursing; 1986:39–54.
18. US Census Bureau, Census 2000 Summary, File 1, Matrices P 3, P 4, PCT 4, PCT 5, PCT 8, and PCT 11.
19. Flynn BC, Dennis L. Health promotion through healthy cities. In Stanhope M, Lancaster J, eds. *Community Health Nursing: Promoting Health of Aggregates, Families, and Individuals.* 4th ed. St. Louis: Mosby; 1996:289–314.
20. Fetterman DM. *Ethnography Step by Step.* Newbury Park, Calif: Sage; 1989.
21. Spradley JP. *The Ethnographic Interview.* Fort Worth, Tex: Harcourt Brace Jovanovich College Publishers; 1979.
22. Austin DE. Cultural knowledge and the cognitive map. *Pract Anthropol.* 1998;20:21–24.
23. Collier J. Evaluating visual data. In: Wagner J, ed. *Images of Information: Still Photography in the Social Sciences.* Beverly Hills, Calif: Sage; 1979:161–169.
24. Patton MQ. *Qualitative Research and Evaluation Methods.* 2nd ed. Newbury Park, Calif: Sage; 1990.
25. van Manen M. *Researching Lived Experience.* New York: State University of New York Press; 1990.
26. Lincoln YS, Guba ED. *Naturalistic Inquiry.* Beverly Hills, Calif: Sage; 1985.
27. Geertz C. *The Interpretation of Cultures.* New York: Basic Books; 1973.
28. Putnam RD. Bowling alone: America's declining social capital. *J Democracy.* 1995;6:65–78.
29. Gittell R, Vidal A. *Community Organizing: Building Social Capital as a Development Strategy.* Thousand Oaks, Calif: Sage; 1998.
30. Schwab M, Syme L. On paradigms, community participation, and the future of public health. *Am J Public Health.* 1997;87:2049–2052.

Copyright © 2006. Lippincott Williams & Wilkins. *Study Guide to Accompany Essentials of Nursing Research,* by Denise F. Polit and Cheryl Tatano Beck.

31. Freire P. *Pedagogy of the Oppressed*. New York: Continuum Publishing Company; 1970.
32. Israel BA, Checkoway B, Schulz A, Zimmerman M. Health education and community empowerment: conceptualizing and measuring perceptions of individual organizational and community control. *Health Educ Q*. 1994;21:149–170.
33. Durch JS, Bailey LA, Stoto MA, eds. *Improving Health in the Community A Role for Performance Measuring*. Washington, DC: National Academy Press; 1997.

Copyright © 2006. Lippincott Williams & Wilkins. *Study Guide to Accompany Essentials of Nursing Research*, by Denise F. Polit and Cheryl Tatano Beck.

A RANDOMIZED CONTROL TRIAL OF NURSING-BASED CASE MANAGEMENT FOR PATIENTS WITH CHRONIC OBSTRUCTIVE PULMONARY DISEASE

Elizabeth Egan, RN, MHSc • Alexandra Clavarino, PhD, BA • Letitia Burridge, RN, MPH • Margaret Teuwen, RN, BScN • Elizabeth White, RN, MSc

This study assessed the impact of a randomized trial of nursing-based case management for patients with chronic obstructive pulmonary disease, their caregivers, and nursing and medical staff. Sixty-six patients were matched by FEV_1 on admission to hospital, and randomized into an intervention or control group. Intervention group patients reported significantly less anxiety at 1 month postdischarge; however, this effect was not sustained. There was little difference between groups in terms of unplanned readmissions, depression, symptoms, support, and subjective well being. Interviews with patients and caregivers found that the case management improved access to resources and staff-patient communication. Interviews with nursing and medical staff found that case management improved communication between staff and enhanced patient care.

■ **Key Words:** Case management; Pulmonary Disease, Chronic Obstructive; Quality of life.

Chronic Obstructive Pulmonary Disease (COPD) is a prevalent, complex, and costly condition to manage.[1,2] It is a progressive and rarely reversible disease[3] in which dyspnea, chronic fatigue, anxiety, and depression are common features.[4,5,6] The physical and social restrictions associated with the condition can have a strong combined influence on patients' functional status and quality of life.[7,8,4] Achieving quality of life for patients

Reprinted with permission from *Lippincott's Case Management* 2002; 7[5]: 170–179.

Copyright © 2006. Lippincott Williams & Wilkins. *Study Guide to Accompany Essentials of Nursing Research*, by Denise F. Polit and Cheryl Tatano Beck.

with COPD entails collaboration among multiple healthcare providers[9,10] and both patient and caregiver. Because no single healthcare provider assumes overall responsibility for the patient,[11] patients or family members are often left to coordinate their care with limited resources and little knowledge of how to access the necessary services within the complexities of the current healthcare system. As a result, service delivery is often fragmented. This can confuse the patient and caregiver and may compromise the achievement of desired healthcare outcomes.

Case management offers an appropriate alternative approach to the management of COPD.[1] As a formal disease management program, it addresses the need for individualized care associated with the experience of COPD. The case manager's (CM) ideal role is to plan and coordinate the delivery of quality services to meet individual patients' needs, reducing the fragmentation of care delivery and improving the quality of life of patients with complex needs.[12] Because case management and nursing practice focus on individual patients' needs and quality of life, specialist nursing staff are well situated to act as CMs.[13] However, in practice, case management has evolved into a focus that is both economic and clinical. The literature indicates an increasing emphasis on the economic side rather than the clinical approach to individual care.[14,15] The few studies that have evaluated the implementation of case management for patients with COPD focus primarily on economic outcomes, rather than patient outcomes.[16,17,18] The results of these studies suggest that case management can reduce the number of days in hospital for patients experiencing recurrent admissions.[16] Less attention has been given to understanding patient-focused outcomes. The purpose of this study was to compare the effect of a brief nursing-based case management intervention with that of normal care for patients hospitalized with COPD.

▪ Method

The study design was a randomized controlled trial. Consecutive patients who were admitted with COPD to a major private hospital in Brisbane, Australia, between July 1999 and September 2000, and who met the following eligibility criteria were invited to participate in the study:

- Aged 18 years or older.
- History of chronic bronchitis (with infection), emphysema, chronic airway obstruction, chronic asthma, or a combination of these.
- Forced Expiratory Volume (FEV_1) on admission prior to initializing intravenous medications to determine severity of disease. This resulted in categories of mild/moderate or severe disease, as determined by the admitting respiratory physician in accordance with the American Thoracic Society guidelines: mild or moderate disease: lung functioning 35% to 50% of predicted value, based on the FEV_1; severe disease: lung functioning was below 35% of predicted value, based on FEV_1.
- Cognitive function at time of entry to the study was adequate to understand and complete a questionnaire.
- Admission to a respiratory unit bed within 72 hours of admission to hospital.
- Informed consent was obtained in writing.

Copyright © 2006. Lippincott Williams & Wilkins. *Study Guide to Accompany Essentials of Nursing Research*, by Denise F. Polit and Cheryl Tatano Beck.

RANDOMIZATION

Patients were first stratified into two groups on the basis of their lung function: mild/moderate and severe. Random number tables were then used as a basis for allocating patients into either the intervention or the control groups.

The study received ethical clearance from the participating hospital.

THE CASE MANAGEMENT INTERVENTION

The CM's position was implemented on a trial basis for this project. The RN in this position held postgraduate qualifications in asthma education, as well as extensive experience in respiratory and thoracic nursing. Following the patient's admission, the CM conducted a comprehensive nursing assessment for patients assigned to the intervention group to identify physical, psychological, social, spiritual, and resource needs. The CM cocoordinated the patient's care during hospitalization utilizing a clinical path, and facilitated ongoing communication between the patient, the caregiver (if there was one), and all healthcare professionals participating in the patient's care. These included medical, nursing, and allied health personnel. The CM provided education for the patient and caregiver on managing the disease, medications, rehabilitation, and available community services, and arranged discharge planning. Following discharge the CM provided ongoing support and acted as a referral point for community services for the patient and caregiver. The CM ensured that planned outcomes were achieved through phone calls to the patient and caregiver on a regular basis. Components of the 6-week intervention are summarized in Table 1.

All patients received nursing assessments and were commenced on standardized clinical paths during admission. However, as Table 1 demonstrates, patients in the intervention group received a comprehensive nursing assessment by the CM who also coordinated their care during hospitalization, conducted a case conference as part of discharge planning for intervention patients, and provided follow-up care at 1 week and 6 weeks post-discharge. Patients in the control group received normal care. This meant that they had no contact with the CM, no case conferences, and no postdischarge follow-up by nursing staff from the respiratory unit.

■ Data Collection

Quantitative and qualitative data were obtained from patients, nursing staff, and allied health staff directly involved with patients' care. Face-to-face interviews were conducted with the respiratory physicians managing the care of all participants (control and intervention).

OUTCOME MEASURES

Patients

The measurements for patients were selected based on key outcomes specific to COPD, including respiratory distress, social support, anxiety, depression, and subjective well being. Both generic and disease specific scales were used.

Copyright © 2006. Lippincott Williams & Wilkins. *Study Guide to Accompany Essentials of Nursing Research*, by Denise F. Polit and Cheryl Tatano Beck.

TABLE 1 Comparison of Care Provided to Control and Intervention Groups

Group	T1 Admission	During Hospitalization	1 Week Post-discharge	T2 1 Month Post-discharge	6 Weeks Post-discharge	T3 3 Months Post-discharge
INTERVENTION						
Nursing Assessment and Review—Case Manager	•	•				
St George Respiratory Questionnaire	•			•		•
Social Support Survey	•			•		•
Hospital Anxiety & Depression Scale	•			•		•
Subjective Well-Being Scale	•			•		•
COPD Clinical Path	•	•				
Discharge Planning	•	•				
Coordinated Care—Case Manager	•	•	•		•	
CONTROL						
Nursing Assessment and Review—Case Manager	•					
St George Respiratory Questionnaire	•			•		•
Social Support Survey	•			•		•
Hospital Anxiety & Depression Scale	•			•		•
Subjective Well-Being Scale	•			•		•
COPD Clinical Path	•	•				
Discharge Planning	•	•				
Coordinated Care—Case Manager	•					

COPD, chronic obstructive pulmonary disease.

Copyright © 2006. Lippincott Williams & Wilkins. *Study Guide to Accompany Essentials of Nursing Research*, by Denise F. Polit and Cheryl Tatano Beck.

The St Georges Respiratory Questionnaire

The St Georges Respiratory Questionnaire (SGRQ)[19] has been widely used to measure health-related quality of life in patients with chronic respiratory disease. The SGRQ consists of 50 items, with 76 responses that produce three domain scores and one overall score. The 3 domains are: the frequency and severity of respiratory symptoms; activities that cause or are limited by breathlessness; and impacts, which relates to social functioning and psychological disturbances resulting from airways disease. The symptoms are scored on a 5-point Likert scale, while activity and impacts are dichotomous (yes/no) items. The 'Total' score summarizes the impact of the disease on overall health status. Scores are expressed as a proportion of overall impairment, in which "0" represents the best possible health status and "100" the worst possible health status.

The Social Support Survey

The Social Support Survey,[20] a measure designed specifically for use with chronically ill populations, was used to measure availability of social support across 4 dimensions of social support: tangible, affectionate, positive social interaction, and emotional/informational support. A higher score for an individual scale or for the overall support index indicates more support. Subscale scores are calculated on the average scores for all items in the subscale. The overall support index is calculated as an average of 2 figures: the scores for all 18 items in the 4 subscales, and the score for the additional final item in the survey.

The Hospital Anxiety and Depression Scale

The Hospital Anxiety and Depression Scale (HADS)[21] was developed specifically for use with patients who are physically ill. The scale consists of 2 brief, 7-item subscales of anxiety and depression. Items are summed on each of the 2 subscales. High scores on each scale indicate the presence of problems (non-cases = a score of ≥ 7; doubtful cases = 8–10; definite cases = 11+).

The Subjective Well-Being Scale

The measure of subjective well being comprises 6 items derived from the literature and incorporates both satisfaction[22] and happiness.[23] It has been developed in 2 previous studies.[24,25] All responses were scored on a 4-point Likert scale with higher scores indicating increased well being.

Demographic information was obtained in the first interview with patients and caregivers. Patients' comorbidities and unscheduled hospital readmissions during the study period were documented.

STAFF

Nursing and Allied Health Personnel

Thirty-four nursing and allied health staff, who were directly involved in patient care, were identified as potentially eligible to participate in the study. These comprised all

Copyright © 2006. Lippincott Williams & Wilkins. *Study Guide to Accompany Essentials of Nursing Research*, by Denise F. Polit and Cheryl Tatano Beck.

permanent respiratory unit nursing staff, both full-time and part-time, as well as allied health staff, that is, specialist respiratory physiotherapists and nutritionists. In addition, 3 clinical nurse consultants (CNCs) directly involved in the care of respiratory patients were surveyed. The CNCs were from community liaison, diabetes education, and gerontology.

Respiratory Physicians

Two respiratory physicians were interviewed at the conclusion of the study using a semistructured interview guide. The purpose of these interviews was to obtain physicians' perceptions of the impact of the case management intervention on their patients, as well as any impact this may have had on their communication with the respiratory unit staff. The physicians were also invited to express their views regarding potential future developments in respiratory care arising out of the study.

PROCEDURE

Nursing and Allied Health Staff

Based in interviews with key informants, a questionnaire was developed to obtain information from staff members regarding the impact of case management upon their working lives and upon patient care and outcomes in general. The questionnaire comprised 16 structured questions measured on a 4-point Likert scale with higher scores indicating greater impact. The self-completed questionnaire was mailed to all eligible staff. Nonresponders were followed up after 2 weeks. Data collection was carried out by a Research Assistant with postgraduate qualifications in psychology.

■ Data Analysis

STATISTICAL METHODS

Quantitative data were analyzed using SPSS. First, demographic and baseline data from the two patient groups were summarized to determine the comparability of the two groups. Descriptive statistics were calculated for the two patient groups separately for each of the data collection points, to observe trends over time in the main outcome measures. As the data were not normally distributed, the non-parametric Wilcoxon matched pairs signed ranks test was used for within group comparisons and the Mann-Whitney test was used to compare groups at each time point.

QUALITATIVE ANALYSIS: PATIENTS

A sub-group of eighteen patients and their caregivers, comprising eight couples and two patients without caregivers, were interviewed in depth regarding their experiences during

Copyright © 2006. Lippincott Williams & Wilkins. *Study Guide to Accompany Essentials of Nursing Research,* by Denise F. Polit and Cheryl Tatano Beck.

the study period. These interviews were semi-structured and focused on issues associated with patient and caregiver satisfaction with care. Participants were selected to maximize variability and to represent both intervention and control groups. Patients and caregivers were interviewed at home. All interviews, including those with the respiratory physicians were audiotaped then transcribed and coded to identify recurring themes and patterns.

■ Results

Sixty-six participants were recruited into the study, and were allocated to either the intervention or control group as shown in Table 2. Because of the small sample size, it was decided to aggregate stratified data, and to simply compare outcomes for the intervention and control groups.

Only two patients (3%) refused to participate. A further 61 potentially eligible patients were excluded from the study. Of these 57% were excluded because no FEV_1 was performed or they were unable to be transferred to a respiratory unit bed within 72 hours of admission. A further 25% were excluded as they had been previously case-managed, and the remainder were excluded for reasons including frail condition and cognitive impairment.

DEMOGRAPHIC CHARACTERISTICS OF THE PATIENTS

Almost two-thirds of the control group were males, and females were similarly represented in the intervention group. This is the only variable with a statistically significant difference between intervention and control groups. As Table 3 demonstrates, no other significant differences were identified between groups regarding demographic characteristics, suggesting that randomization was effective.

Most respondents had completed at least grade 10 level of education, were outside the workforce, married or living with a partner and were Australian born. Most reported medium to high levels of income and were primarily Anglican or Catholic. Patient numbers declined slightly at each time interval, with a total of 24% lost from the control group, compared with 15% from the intervention group. These losses were due to patient deaths (n = 5) and withdrawals (n = 8).

TABLE 2 Participants by Group and Severity of Disease

	Control	Intervention	Total
Severe	19	19	38
Mild/Moderate	14	14	28
Total	33	33	66

Copyright © 2006. Lippincott Williams & Wilkins. *Study Guide to Accompany Essentials of Nursing Research*, by Denise F. Polit and Cheryl Tatano Beck.

TABLE 3 Demographic Characteristics of Participants

Characteristics		Control (n = 33)		Intervention (n = 33)	
Mean Age		67.8		67.2	
		$P = 0.789$			
Gender	Male	20	60%	12	36%
	Female	13	40%	21	64%
	$P = 0.049$				
Level of Education	Completed primary	7	21%	5	15%
	Completed year 10	12	36%	12	36%
	Completed year 12	5	15%	6	18%
	Trade/apprenticeship/ certificate/diploma	5	15%	6	18%
	Bachelor degree/higher	4	13%	4	13%
	$P = 0.989$				
Employment Status	In workforce	3	9%	5	15%
	Outside workforce	30	91%	28	85%
	$P = 0.621$				
Marital Status	Married/living with partner	24	73%	21	64%
	Not married or living with partner	9	27%	12	36%
	$P = 0.158$				
Level of Income	Up to $20,000	8	26%	10	31%
	$20,001 to 40,000	11	35%	14	44%
	>$40,000	12	39%	8	25%
	$P = 0.077$				
Country of Birth	Australia	26	87%	31	94%
	Other	4	13%	2	6%
	$P = 0.366$				
Religion	Anglican	7	23%	11	38%
	Catholic	8	28%	9	31%
	Other	6	21%	4	14%
	None	8	28%	5	17%
	$P = 0.426$				
Patient has a Caregiver	Yes	26	78.8%	24	72.7%
	$P = 0.567$				

Copyright © 2006. Lippincott Williams & Wilkins. *Study Guide to Accompany Essentials of Nursing Research*, by Denise F. Polit and Cheryl Tatano Beck.

CHANGE OVER TIME

Tables 4 and 5 show the changes that occurred in key outcome variables between admission (T1) and one month post-discharge (T2), and between one (T2) and three months post-discharge (T3). All median changes refer to the intervals between T1 and T2 or T2 and T3. The final column contains the p-value for the unpaired Mann-Whitney test with a null hypothesis that the change in the control group equals the change in the intervention group.

Both groups reported an improvement in symptoms between admission and one month post discharge (see Table 4). This change was considered predictable, in view of the treatment provided during hospitalization. The intervention group reported lower levels of affectionate support, which was significantly different to the control group. The intervention group experienced a significant improvement in the level of anxiety between hospitalization and one-month post discharge, but this was not significantly different from the control group. The improvement in symptoms, which occurred between T1 and T2, was not sustained to T3 for either group. The control group reported lower levels of activity between T2 and T3. No other significant differences were identified either within or between groups.

UNSCHEDULED HOSPITAL READMISSIONS

There were no significant differences between groups regarding unscheduled hospital readmissions. The mean number of unscheduled readmits for the intervention group patients was 2.1 (range 10 (n = 1) to 5 (n = 2)) and for control group patients was 2.6 (range 1 (n = 11) to 6 (n = 3)).

QUALITATIVE ANALYSIS: PATIENTS

Based on the qualitative interviews, all patients were very satisfied with their care in hospital. Participants in the control group who had extensive family and medical support, particularly from a general practitioner, appeared to be quite satisfied with their access to community services. For patients in the control group without these supports, the situation was much more difficult. As one caregiver explained, 'It is absolutely hopeless.' However, for patients in the intervention group, ongoing contact with the CM proved to be very beneficial, particularly in terms of improving communication between health care personnel and patients. As one patient commented, "On the last visit I became more involved with (the CM) and it was good to know that she cared, but perhaps before that...sometimes when you came home you were just as bad as when you went in, but you weren't—you just felt it. But (the CM) kept on your hammer all the time . . . So I think that...it will give some peace of mind to the patients, you know. The big thing is to know what is happening."

A number of intervention group patients and caregivers also made the point that case management facilitated access to resources and equipment which they would never otherwise have accessed.

Copyright © 2006. Lippincott Williams & Wilkins. *Study Guide to Accompany Essentials of Nursing Research*, by Denise F. Polit and Cheryl Tatano Beck.

TABLE 4 Differences in Patients' Experiences, Between T1 (Baseline) and T2 (1 Month Postdischarge)

| | Intervention (I) | | | Control (C) | | | I vs C |
	n	Median change	P	n	Median change	P	P
St G–Symptoms	27	−17.5	0.01	25	−9.3	0.001	0.384
St G–Activities	25	0	0.895	26	0.4	0.746	0.727
St G–Impacts	26	−0.2	0.647	23	−0.9	0.515	0.849
St G–Total	22	−1.6	0.420	24	−1.5	0.149	0.621
Tangible Support	25	0	0.422	26	0	0.460	0.523
Affectionate Support	23	−6.7	0.004	26	0	0.660	0.034
Positive Social Intervention	23	0	0.174	25	0	0.814	0.595
Emotional Support	24	0	0.746	26	0	0.735	0.907
HADS Anxiety	25	−1.0	0.017	26	−2.5	0.059	0.437
HADS Depression	26	0.5	0.892	27	−1	0.402	0.383
Total SWB	27	2.8	0.744	27	−2.8	0.450	0.416

St. G, St. George; SWB, Subjective Well Being; HADS, Hospital Anxiety and Depression Scale.

Copyright © 2006. Lippincott Williams & Wilkins. *Study Guide to Accompany Essentials of Nursing Research*, by Denise F. Polit and Cheryl Tatano Beck.

TABLE 5 Differences in Patients' Experiences, Between T2 (1 Month Postdischarge) and T3 (3 Months Postdischarge)

	Intervention (I)			Control (C)			I vs C
	n	Median Change	P	n	Median Change	P	P
St G–Symptoms	26	2.0	0.824	22	0.5	0.987	0.959
St G–Activities	24	0	1.0	20	-6.4	0.0003	0.01
St G–Impacts	26	2.5	0.777	20	-1.5	0.245	0.432
St G–Total	22	0.6	0.766	19	-3.2	0.123	0.367
Tangible Support	26	-2.5	0.864	22	-5.0	0.714	0.723
Affectionate Support	24	10.0	0.228	22	0	0.796	0.323
Positive Social Intervention	24	0.0	0.602	22	-2.5	0.434	0.756
Emotional Support	24	-3.6	0.315	23	2.5	0.199	0.157
HADS Anxiety	24	0	0.986	24	-1.5	0.529	0.764
HADS Depression	24	-0.5	0.930	24	0.5	0.165	0.325
Total SWB	25	-2.8	0.829	24	0	0.189	0.268

St G, St. George; SWB, Subjective Well Being; HADS, Hospital Anxiety and Depression Scale.

Copyright © 2006. Lippincott Williams & Wilkins. *Study Guide to Accompany Essentials of Nursing Research*, by Denise F. Polit and Cheryl Tatano Beck.

(The CM) made me aware of things that were available that I didn't bother to want to know about before. [Patient]

    (The CM) helped me organize (a nebuliser); she pointed out a lot of things to me, different things that should be done (for the patient). [Caregiver].

NURSING AND ALLIED HEALTH PERSONNEL

Questionnaires were distributed to 30 of the 34 personnel directly involved in patient care. (Four were on leave during the survey). A total of 22 (65%) questionnaires were returned. 16 (73%) respondents were Respiratory Unit nurses; 3 (13.5%) were allied health (physiotherapists) and 3 (13.5%) were clinical nurse consultants in the following specialties: community liaison, gerontology and diabetes education. All but 2 respondents (9.1%) were female. Of the 16 who reported their age, 4 were under 30 years; 2 were aged between 30 and 39 years; 6 were between 40 and 49 years and the remainder were aged 50 years or older.

Personnel were asked to rank the impact of case management on a number of items, and their responses are presented in Table 6.

Respondents reported at least some improvement in discharge planning, coordination of resources outside the hospital and coordination of care within the hospital. Approximately two-thirds of respondents reported a positive impact on human resources by improving working relationships, ward efficiency, and patient care. More than half of those surveyed felt that case management decreased their workload and stress level, while increasing both their involvement and time spent in patient care. Approximately two-thirds of respondents reported at least some improvement in patient-focused issues such as patients' knowledge of their disease, compliance with their prescribed regimes, and disease self-management. Most were confident that patient outcomes would be improved.

Nursing and allied health staff found the implementation of case management beneficial, not only to patients but also to ward operation. Most reported improvements in patient care, and also in patients' compliance, knowledge and management of their disease. The CM facilitated communication within the ward, improved the coordination of care, and acted as a resource person for ward personnel.

Personnel were also invited to supplement their questionnaire responses with other comments. Without exception, the comments highlighted the positive impact of case management on patient care, personnel and on the hospital. A number of respondents commented on the '*improved quality of patient care*' since the introduction of a CM. Personnel also reported that feedback from patients had been positive, because . . . *patients are pleased, and find it a great help . . . to be able to contact and speak with the person they have come to know and rely on with follow-up care, with just a phone call.*

Staff believed that CMs/specialist nurses were needed for the '*whole hospital,*' not simply one unit. One respondent said that *this professional approach to discharge care should be implemented on every ward, to lessen the anxiety of a patient and family on his/her discharge from the ward.*

One Clinical Nurse Consultant (CNC) responsible for discharge planning reported far fewer referrals from the respiratory unit, suggesting that '*planning must be happening.*'

Copyright © 2006. Lippincott Williams & Wilkins. *Study Guide to Accompany Essentials of Nursing Research*, by Denise F. Polit and Cheryl Tatano Beck.

TABLE 6 Nursing and Allied Health Staff: Satisfaction With the Impact of Case Management

Item	Not at all/ A Little N (%)	Somewhat/ Quite a Lot N (%)	Unsure N (%)
1 Reduction in unplanned admissions	6 (27.2)	8 (36.4)	8 (36.4)
2 Improved discharge planning	1 (4.5)	20 (91.0)	1 (4.5)
3 Reduction in average length of patient stay	4 (18.1)	12 (54.6)	6 (27.3)
4 Improved coordination of resources outside hospital	—	22 (100)	—
5 Improved patient compliance with prescribed regimes	1 (4.5)	18 (81.8)	3 (13.6)
6 Improved coordination of care within hospital	1 (4.5)	21 (95.4)	—
7 Improved cohesiveness of staff relationships	3 (13.6)	16 (72.7)	3 (13.6)
8 Reduction in personal workload	7 (33.3)	12 (57.2)	2 (9.5)
9 Reduction in the level of stress felt	6 (27.2)	14 (63.6)	2 (9.1)
10 Increased time available for patient care	6 (27.3)	13 (59.1)	3 (13.6)
11 Increased sense of involvement in patient care	7 (31.8)	12 (54.5)	3 (13.6)
12 Improved patient care	2 (9.1)	19 (86.3)	1 (4.5)
13 Improved patient outcomes	2 (9.1)	17 (77.3)	3 (13.6)
14 Improved efficiency of the ward	2 (9.1)	18 (81.8)	2 (9.1)
15 Improved patients' knowledge of their disease	—	20 (90.9)	2 (9.1)
16 Improved patients' management of their disease	2 (9.1)	17 (77.2)	3 (13.6)

Not all percentages total 100% due to rounding.

Another CNC reported receiving more referrals about self-care education, which she believed '*is excellent care for the patient.*'

COMMENTS FROM PHYSICIANS

Although the physicians noticed no differences between patients receiving case management and those who did not, they valued having a CM to contact. One commented,

> I have found it really helpful having (the CM) who has been very interested in particular patients and who we have been able to call (on). . .

The physicians believed that the CM enhanced ward communication, specifically '*with [admitting respiratory physician]s and nursing staff,*' and fulfilled the role of clinical resource person for personnel. As one respondent commented, the CM '*improved*

Copyright © 2006. Lippincott Williams & Wilkins. *Study Guide to Accompany Essentials of Nursing Research*, by Denise F. Polit and Cheryl Tatano Beck.

nursing staff's knowledge of [the] disease process, management of acute episodes and treatment regimes.'

■ Discussion

This is one of the first studies that set out to evaluate a nurse based case management intervention to help COPD patients manage their disease and access to services. Little difference was found between the control and intervention groups in terms of the key outcome variables: anxiety, depression, symptoms, support and subjective well-being. While some improvement was noted in levels of intervention group anxiety at one month, the effect was not sustained. This was possibly due to the brief nature of the intervention. A more intensive follow-up may overcome this problem as intensive case management has been found to enhance patient outcomes in studies of mental health,[26] particularly for patients who are frequently hospitalized.[27] A longer time-frame for the follow-up may also have shown significant differences. The intervention had a positive impact on the psychological well-being of patients, but the effect diminished over time, suggesting that patients need ongoing support. Based on studies with mental health patients a minimum follow-up time of twelve months has been recommended with few effects discernible before one year.[25] Similarly, intervention group patients reported a decline in levels of affectionate support post-discharge, possibly reflecting the loss of close contact with the CM. This may also reflect the fact that more intervention patients than controls were without a caregiver. Although this difference was not statistically significant, it is evident from the qualitative data that the CM was seen by a number of patients as having a caring role.

In-depth interviews revealed considerable differences between groups particularly in relation to the high value placed on case management by intervention group participants. Quantitative and qualitative data indicated that the majority of nursing and medical staff found case management beneficial to patients, the ward and the hospital particularly in relation to facilitating staff-patient communication and the implementation of planned care.

This study has some limitations. A number of potentially eligible patients were not invited into the study or were excluded because they were admitted to other wards before being transferred to the respiratory unit, and because spirometry was not completed upon admission. However, there is no reason to believe that these patients would differ from patients who were enrolled, in ways relevant to this study. Given the small sample size, it was not possible to identify significant differences between the two strata comprising each group. Differences in severity of disease need to be explored in further studies.

■ Conclusion

The study set out to evaluate a brief case management intervention for patients with COPD. Further research is recommended to investigate the impact on key outcomes of a rehabilitation and education program for COPD patients.

Copyright © 2006. Lippincott Williams & Wilkins. *Study Guide to Accompany Essentials of Nursing Research*, by Denise F. Polit and Cheryl Tatano Beck.

The study provided evidence to suggest that Case Management is an effective model of care for COPD patients. The recommendation has been made that a permanent CM be appointed to the respiratory unit to facilitate patient care during hospitalization and following discharge. Based on this study, the specific qualifications for this person would include:

- advanced clinical knowledge in the specialty area
- well-developed communication and negotiation skills
- the ability to work as a member of a multidisciplinary team
- the ability to advocate on behalf of the patient/family
- education expertise—patient/family and staff
- a knowledge of outcomes management.

The hospital involved in this study is currently developing a similar approach to the care of oncology and stroke patients.

To successfully introduce such a program it is essential to have the support of all levels of hospital administration. It is also necessary to involve medical staff who are willing to contribute to planning and development.

The study highlighted the necessity for improved communication between the hospital and existing community service providers. As the majority of care delivery for this group of patients occurs within the community setting, a successful program must incorporate an education component which includes the community aspects of care. The CM must develop channels of communication, both formal and informal, between patient/family, the hospital and community service providers.

Address correspondence and reprint requests to: Elizabeth Egan, Clinical Nurse Consultant, Continuing Care, The Wesley Hospital, PO Box 499, Toowong. Qld. 4066, Australia (e-mail: eegan@wesley.com.au).

Elizabeth Egan has extensive experience in oncology nursing and an interest in improving the management and treatment for people with chronic disease. She gained post graduate qualification in the field of health education and currently is working in the area of hospital/community interface, The Wesley Hospital, Brisbane, Australia.

Dr Alexandra Clavarino has a PhD in Sociology from The University of Queensland and has extensive experience teaching qualitative and quantitative research methods. With over ten years' experience in the quality of life of cancer patients, her research interests include cancer and quality of life issues, women's and rural health, and patient services. He currently works at the Centre for Health Promotion and Cancer Prevention Research, University of Queensland, Brisbane, Australia.

Letitia Burridge has extensive experience in clinical nursing. She is interested in bridging the gap between health care in hospitals and health maintenance in the community. With postgraduate experience in women's health and coping with cancer, her research interests include quality of life in cancer and other chronic illnesses. She currently works at the Centre for Health Promotion and Cancer Prevention Research, University of Queensland, Brisbane, Australia.

Margaret Teuwen has extensive experience in respiratory nursing with an interest in self management of chronic disease. The focus of her current role is the enhancement of patient and caregiver participation in the management of chronic lung disease across the hospital/community continuum. She has post graduate qualification in asthma education and currently works at the Wesley Hospital, Brisbane, Australia.

Elizabeth White has extensive experience in both clinical and management aspects of nursing. She has an MSc (Nursing) from the University of Surrey, UK. Her main research interests include quality of life

Copyright © 2006. Lippincott Williams & Wilkins. *Study Guide to Accompany Essentials of Nursing Research*, by Denise F. Polit and Cheryl Tatano Beck.

issues for persons with chronic illness and the impact of caregiving on the primary family caregiver. She is currently Nursing Director, Medical and Oncology Services The Wesley Hospital, Brisbane.

ACKNOWLEDGMENTS

This study was funded by a grant from The Wesley Research Institute. The authors would also like to thank the following for their assistance with this study: Mrs Lyn Dasey RN, Dr Adrian Barnett, Ms Sue-Ann Carmont.

REFERENCES

1. Alternative approaches to COPD management address needs for individualized care. *Clin Resour Manag.* 2001;2(4):61–63, 49.
2. Australian Institute of Health and Welfare (AIHW). *Australia's Health 2000.* Canberra: AIHW; 2000.
3. Action on Smoking and Health (ASH). *Smoking and Respiratory Disease.* 2001. Available from URL:http://www.ash.org.uk/index.php?
4. Janson C, Bjornsson E, Hetta, J, Boman G. Anxiety and depression in relation to respiratory symptoms and asthma. *Am J Respir Crit Care Med.* 1994;149(4 Pt 1)930–4.
5. Moody L, McCormick K, Williams A. Disease and symptom severity, functional status and quality of life in chronic bronchitis and emphysema (CBE). *J Behav Med.* 1990;13(3):297–306.
6. Light RW, Merrill EJ, Despars JA, Gordon GH, Mutalipassi LR. Prevalence of depression and anxiety in patients with COPD: relationship to functional capacity. *Chest.* 1985;87(1):35–8.
7. Czjkowski SM, McSweeney AJ. The role of psychosocial factors in chronic obstructive pulmonary disease. *Phys Med Rehabil Clin N Am.* 1996;7(2):341–52.
8. Guyatt GH, Bombardier C, Tugwell P. Measuring disease-specific quality of life in clinical trials. *CMAJ.* 1986;134:(8): 889–95.
9. Sabo D. Clinical information system: a "gateway" to the 21st century. *Nurs Adm Q.* 1997;21(3): 68–75.
10. Rabinowitz B, Florian V. Chronic Obstructive Pulmonary Disease - psycho-social issues and treatment goals. *Soc Work Health Care.* 1992;16(4):69–86.
11. Faherty B. Case Management: The latest buzzword: What it is and what it isn't. *Caring.* 1990;9(7):20–2.
12. Mayer GG. Case management as a mindset. *Qual Manag Health Care.* 1996;5(1):7–16.
13. Newman MA. Toward an integrative model of professional practice. *J Prof Nurs.* 1990;6(3):167–73.
14. Yarmo D, McDonald M. Wenborn J. Case management at Warringal Private Hospital: challenges of development, implementation and evaluation. *Aust Health Rev.* 1998;21(4):221–37.
15. Smith, MC. Case management and nursing theory-based practice. *Nurs Sci Q.* 1993;6(1):8–9.
16. Poole PJ, Chase B, Frankel A. Black PN. Case management may reduce length of hospital stay in patients with recurrent admissions for chronic obstructive pulmonary disease. *Respirology.* 2001;6(1):37–42.
17. Lagoe RJ, Noetscher CM, Murphy ME. Combined benchmarking of hospital outcomes and utilization. *Nurs Econ.* 2000;18(2):63–70.
18. COPD pathway cuts costs per case by $900. *Hosp Case Manag.* 1997;5(9):156–158.
19. Jones PW, Quirk FH, Baveystock CM. The St George's Respiratory Questionnaire. *Respir Med.* 1991;85 Suppl B:25–31, Discussion:33–7.
20. Sherbourne CD, Stewart AL. The MOS Social Support Survey. *Soc Sci Med.* 1991;32(6):705–14.
21. Zigmond AS, Snaith RP. The Hospital Anxiety and Depression Scale. *Acta Psychiatr Scand.* 1983;67(6):361–70.
22. Campbell A, Converse PE, Rodgers WL. *The Quality of American Life Perceptions, Evaluations and Satisfactions.* New York: Russell Sage; 1976.

Copyright © 2006. Lippincott Williams & Wilkins. *Study Guide to Accompany Essentials of Nursing Research,* by Denise F. Polit and Cheryl Tatano Beck.

23. Bradburn N. *The Structure of Psychological Well-Being*. Chicago: Aldine; 1969.
24. Clavarino AM. Dying-From Experience. [PhD thesis]. Queensland, Australia: University of Queensland; 1997.
25. Yates P. The Use of Alternative Therapies by People With Metastatic Cancer: A Multivariate Analysis. [Masters thesis]. Department of Anthropology and Sociology. Queensland, Australia: University of Queensland; 1991.
26. Preston NJ, Fazio S. Establishing the efficacy and cost effectiveness of community intensive case management of long-term mentally ill: a matched control group study. *Aust N Z J Psychiatry*. 2000;34(1):114–21.
27. Chamberlain R, Rapp, CA. (1991) A decade of case management: a methodological review of outcome research. *Community Ment Health J*. 1991;27(3):171–88.

Copyright © 2006. Lippincott Williams & Wilkins. *Study Guide to Accompany Essentials of Nursing Research*, by Denise F. Polit and Cheryl Tatano Beck.

THE EFFECTIVENESS OF TAI CHI EXERCISE IN IMPROVING AEROBIC CAPACITY

A Meta-Analysis

Ruth E. Taylor-Piliae, RN, CNS, MN

Erika S. Froelicher, RN, MPH, PhD, FAAN

- **Purpose:** Meta-analysis involves the integration of several studies with small sample sizes, enabling the investigator to summarize research results into useful clinical information. Tai Chi exercise has recently gained the attention of Western researchers as a potential form of aerobic exercise. A goal of this meta-analysis was to estimate the effect of Tai Chi exercise on aerobic capacity.
- **Methods:** A computerized search of 7 databases was done using key words and all languages. Sixteen study elements were critically appraised to determine study quality. D-STAT software was used to calculate the standardized mean differences (ES_{sm}) and the 95% confidence intervals (CI), using means and standard deviations (SD) reported on aerobic capacity expressed as peak oxygen uptake ($\dot{V}O_2$ peak) ($mL \cdot kg^{-1} \cdot min^{-1}$).
- **Results:** Of 441 citations obtained, only 7 focused on aerobic capacity in response to Tai Chi exercise (4 experimental and 3 cross-sectional). Older adults including those with heart disease participated ($n = 344$ subjects); on average men were aged 55.7 years (SD = 12.7) and women 60.7 years (SD = 6.2). Study quality scores ranged from 22 to 28 (mean = 25.1, SD = 2.0). Average effect size for the cross-sectional studies was large and statistically significant ($ES_{sm} = 1.01$; CI = +0.37, +1.66), while in the experimental studies the average effect size was small and not significant ($ES_{sm} = 0.33$; CI = −0.41, +1.07). Effect sizes of aerobic capacity in women ($ES_{sm} = 0.83$; CI = −0.43, +2.09) were greater than those for men ($ES_{sm} = 0.65$; CI = −0.04, +1.34), though not statistically significant. Aerobic capacity was higher in subjects performing classical Yang style (108 postures) Tai Chi ($ES_{sm} = 1.10$; CI = +0.82, +1.38), a 52-week Tai Chi

---

Reprinted with permission from *Journal of Cardiovascular Nursing* 2004; 19[1]: 48–57.

Copyright © 2006. Lippincott Williams & Wilkins. *Study Guide to Accompany Essentials of Nursing Research,* by Denise F. Polit and Cheryl Tatano Beck.

exercise intervention (ES_{sm} = 0.94; C = +0.06, +1.81), compared with sedentary subjects (ES_{sm} = 0.80; CI = +0.19, +1.41).

- **Conclusions**: This meta-analysis suggests that Tai Chi may be an additional form of aerobic exercise. The greatest benefit was seen from the classical Yang style of Tai Chi exercise when performed for 1-year by sedentary adults with an initial low level of physical activity habits. Recommendations for future research are provided and the effect sizes generated provide information needed for sample size calculations. Randomized clinical trials in diverse populations, including those with chronic diseases, would expand the current knowledge about the effect of Tai Chi on aerobic capacity.
- **Key Words**: aerobic capacity, meta-analysis, oxygen consumption, Tai Chi

Tai Chi exercise, though practiced in China for hundreds of years, has only recently gained the interest of researchers in Western countries as an alternative form of exercise.[1-3] Recently, improvements in cardiorespiratory function,[4-6] balance,[7-9] muscular strength,[10-12] flexibility,[5,13,14] relaxation[15,16] and mood state[15,17-19] have been associated with Tai Chi. Additionally, reduction in blood pressure,[3,20] and improvement in aerobic capacity[2] in patients with heart disease have been reported. Tai Chi requires no special facility or expensive equipment and can be performed either individually or in groups. Tai Chi movements are suited for persons of all ages, regardless of previous exercise experience and aerobic capacity.[14,21] Tai Chi is a low impact, low to moderate intensity exercise incorporating elements of balance, strength, flexibility, relaxation, and body alignment. Features of Tai Chi exercise include weight-shifting between right and left legs, knee flexion, straight and extended head and trunk, rotation, and asymmetrical diagonal arm and leg movements with bent knees.[22,23] The exercise intensity of Tai Chi is variable and can be adjusted by the height of the postures, duration of the practice session, and training style.[22,23] Tai Chi is performed in a semisquat position. A high-squat posture and short-training session are well suited for deconditioned persons, including those with heart disease and older adults.[22,23] The exercise intensity of Tai Chi, height of the postures, and duration are all likely to affect overall improvements in aerobic capacity. However, there is a paucity of literature on the aerobic benefits of Tai Chi exercise.

Lan and colleagues[22] reported the exercise intensity during performance of the classical Yang style among experienced Tai Chi practitioners to be at 55% of the subjects' peak oxygen uptake. Zhuo and colleagues[24] reported the estimated energy costs of performing the classical Yang style of Tai Chi to be 4.1 metabolic equivalents (METs), with work intensity not exceeding 50% of an individual's maximum oxygen uptake. Schneider and Leung[25] reported that the exercise intensity of performing Tai Chi was 4.6 METs. Zhuo and colleagues[24] have also reported that the energy cost for performing a simplified form of Tai Chi requires an average of 2.9 METs with a maximum oxygen uptake at less than 40%. Energy requirements for Tai Chi Chih, a simplified form of Tai Chi, were reported by Fontana[26] to range from 1.5 to 2.6 METs,[26] depending on whether the subject was sitting or standing. There seems to be a wide range of exercise intensities associated with Tai Chi performance, ranging from 1.5 to 4.6 METs.

Maximum oxygen consumption ($\dot{V}o_2$ max) is considered the best measure of aerobic capacity and provides important information about cardiorespiratory function.[27,28] $\dot{V}o_2$max is the greatest amount of oxygen a person can take in from inspired air while performing dynamic exercise involving a large part of total muscle mass.[27] $\dot{V}o_2$ max is

Copyright © 2006. Lippincott Williams & Wilkins. *Study Guide to Accompany Essentials of Nursing Research*, by Denise F. Polit and Cheryl Tatano Beck.

considered the gold standard for determining aerobic capacity,[27,28] though not feasible or appropriate for some patient populations. Aerobic capacity is derived from gas exchange during exercise testing and is difficult to obtain in older populations and those with compromised cardiopulmonary functioning. In high risk or diseased populations, it may be more appropriate to obtain $\dot{V}o_2$ peak if symptoms such as angina, deconditioning or other factors prevent subjects from achieving maximum oxygen consumption levels.[27,28] Oxygen consumption derived from $\dot{V}o_2$ peak during exercise testing is most accurate when measured directly from expired gases.[27,28] Another term to express oxygen consumption is *metabolic equivalents*.[27,28] One metabolic equivalent (MET) is a unit of resting oxygen uptake (~3.5 mL of O_2 per kilogram of body weight per minute $[mL \cdot kg^{-1} \cdot min^{-1}]$).[29] In this meta-analysis, $\dot{V}o_2$ peak in $mL \cdot kg^{-1} \cdot min^{-1}$ is used as the measure of aerobic capacity.

The effect of Tai Chi exercise on aerobic capacity is important to know if clinicians want to recommend Tai Chi as an alternative form of aerobic exercise. The majority of the published studies examining cardiorespiratory responses to Tai Chi exercise by measuring aerobic capacity have small sample sizes. A meta-analysis involves the integration of several studies with small or large sample sizes, enabling the investigator to summarize the research results into useful clinical information. Therefore, the purpose of this meta-analysis was to estimate the extent to which Tai Chi exercise affects aerobic capacity.

■ Methods

LITERATURE SEARCH AND STUDY SELECTION

A computerized search of 7 databases (PubMed, CINAHL, Current Contents, Cochrane Library, Digital Dissertations, PsychINFO, and SocAbstracts) was done using key words for the various English language spellings of Tai Chi (eg, Tai Chi, Tai Chi Chuan, Tai Chi Quan, Tai Ji, and Tai Ji Quan). All languages were accepted. A total of 441 citations were obtained. Abstracts of all research studies were reviewed using a study selection form to determine whether subjects were randomly assigned to a Tai Chi exercise intervention or whether a Tai Chi exercise group was compared with another group; and if aerobic capacity was an outcome measure. The following types of articles were rejected: review, commentary, case report, research methodology paper, a reanalysis of data, a meta-analysis, an overview, qualitative research not related to the meta-analysis topic, or if aerobic capacity was not included as an outcome variable. Several articles appeared in more than one database.

Following initial selection criteria, 14 studies and 1 doctoral dissertation were examined in depth to determine whether they met the selection criteria. A total of 8 studies investigated Tai Chi and aerobic capacity and met the inclusion criteria. Four of the articles were experimental studies (2 randomized clinical trials,[19,20] 2 quasi-experimental[2,4]), 3 were cross-sectional studies,[5,25,30] and 1 was a prospective cohort study.[6] In the cross-sectional studies, 2 groups of different subjects were matched on age, gender, and body composition, allowing for adequate group comparisons. The prospective cohort study examined age-related deterioration in aerobic capacity and how Tai Chi may slow

Copyright © 2006. Lippincott Williams & Wilkins. *Study Guide to Accompany Essentials of Nursing Research*, by Denise F. Polit and Cheryl Tatano Beck.

progressive decline. Subjects in the Tai Chi exercise and control groups in the prospective cohort study had statistically significant different baseline $\dot{V}o_2$ scores. Thus, group comparisons at the end of the study were not feasible,[6] and the study was not included in this meta-analysis. Characteristics of the subjects in these studies can be found in Table 1 (experimental) and Table 2 (cross-sectional).

DEVELOPMENT OF STUDY QUALITY SCORING TOOL

A study quality scoring tool was developed on the basis of previous work from Chan and Bartlett.[31] A total of 16 study elements were critically appraised to determine a study quality score. Elements reviewed included study design, sample selection, description of the independent variable (Tai Chi), description of the outcome measure (aerobic capacity), data analyses, and results. The highest possible study quality score was 32; each item had a possible score of 0 to 2 (0 = absent, 1 = partially defined, 2 = clearly defined), with possible scores ranging from 0 to 32. The methodological quality of both experimental and cross-sectional studies could be assessed using this tool. Any study with a quality score below 67% (<21) of the total possible score[31] was eliminated from this analysis.

MEASUREMENTS OF EFFECTS OF TAI CHI EXERCISE ASSESSED

In order to measure the benefits of exercise, the frequency, intensity, duration, type, and preference of exercise need consideration.[27,28] Current recommendations by the American College of Sport Medicine[27,28] include exercise frequency of 3 to 5 days per week, an intensity of either 65% to 90% of maximum heart rate or 50% to 85% of maximal oxygen uptake, duration of 20 to 60 minutes per session, aerobic type activity, and participation in an enjoyable aerobic activity. In very unfit individuals, the exercise intensity based on 55% to 64% of an individual's predicted maximum heart rate may be most suitable.[27,28] Aerobic capacity is influenced by age, weight, gender, exercise habits, genetic factors, and cardiovascular clinical status. Effects of Tai Chi exercise on aerobic capacity in this meta-analysis included study design, gender, physical activity habits, style of Tai Chi exercise, and the duration of the Tai Chi exercise intervention-training period.

DATA ABSTRACTION AND CALCULATION OF EFFECT SIZE

Using the data abstraction form developed for this meta-analysis, information from the 7 studies was abstracted (by Ruth Taylor-Piliae) to record study sample characteristics, the independent variable (Tai Chi), the outcome variable (aerobic capacity, expressed as $\dot{V}o_2$ peak in $mL \cdot kg^{-1} \cdot min^{-1}$), results, and statistical methods. Effect sizes were calculated from the standardized mean differences using means and standard deviations reported on the outcome measure (aerobic capacity).

The standardized mean difference effect size (ES_{sm}), also called d, is a scale-free measure that can contrast results for 2 groups, with continuous underlying distributions.[32,33]

Copyright © 2006. Lippincott Williams & Wilkins. *Study Guide to Accompany Essentials of Nursing Research*, by Denise F. Polit and Cheryl Tatano Beck.

TABLE 1 Experimental Studies

Author/Year	Study Design	Size	Gender	Mean Age in Years (SD)	Tai Chi Style	Length of Intervention	Group	Baseline Mean V̇o₂ peak, mL·kg⁻¹·min⁻¹ (SD)	Follow-up Mean V̇o₂ peak, mL·kg⁻¹·min⁻¹ (SD)	Effect Size	LBCI	UBCI
Brown et al 1995	RCT	11	Male	50.4 (5.7)	Not specified	16 wk	Tai Chi	31.7 (5.1)	30.8 (4.1)	−0.3580	−1.154	+0.4379
		14	Male	50.5 (7.4)			Control (sedentary)	31.9 (5.4)	32.7 (5.8)			
		7	Female	51.5 (8.3)		16 wk	Tai Chi	25.0 (4.4)	23.8 (4.7)	−0.3101	−1.1857	+0.5830
		17	Female	53.6 (9.4)			Control (sedentary)	26.7 (6.0)	25.2 (4.4)			
Lan et al 1998	Quasi-exper	9	Male	65.2 (4.2)	Yang, 108 postures	52 wk	Tai Chi	24.2 (5.2)	28.1 (5.4)	+0.8176	−0.1442	+1.779
		9	Male	66.6 (3.9)			Control (sedentary)	24.0 (4.8)	23.6 (5.0)			
		11	Female	64.9 (4.7)		52 wk	Tai Chi	16.0 (2.5)	19.4 (2.8)	+1.334	+0.3609	+2.307
		9	Female	65.4 (3.8)			Control (sedentary)	15.8 (2.5)	15.6 (2.6)			
Lan et al 1999	Quasi-exper	9	Male	55.7 (7.1)	Yang, 108 postures	52 wk	Tai Chi	26.2 (4.4)	28.9 (5.0)	+0.6572	−0.2469	+1.561
		11	Male	57.2 (7.6)			Control (walking program)	26.0 (3.9)	25.6 (4.6)			
Young et al 1999	RCT	27	Not specified	Not specified	Yang, 13 movements	12 wk	Tai Chi	Not specified	0.97*(4.1)	−0.1598	−0.7105	+0.3909
		24	Not specified	Not specified			Control (aerobic exercise)	Not specified	1.64* (4.1)			

Note: RCT denotes randomized clinical trial; Quasi-exper, quasi-experimental study; WK, week; LBCI, lower bound confidence interval; and UBCI; upper bound confidence interval. Effect size is not significant if 0 is included in the confidence interval.
*Mean change in aerobic capacity.

Copyright © 2006. LIPPINCOTT WILLIAMS & WILKINS. *Study Guide to Accompany Essentials of Nursing Research*, by Denise F. Polit and Cheryl Tatano Beck.

TABLE 2 Cross-Sectional Studies*

Author/Year	Study Design	Size	Gender	Mean Age in Years (SD)	Group	Tai Chi Style	Mean $\dot{V}o_2$ peak, $mL \cdot kg^{-1} \cdot min^{-1}$ (SD)	Effect Size	LBCI	UBCI
Schneider et al 1991	Cross-sectional	10	Male	35.5 (3.9)	Tai Chi	Not specified	44.3 (6.6)	+0.1571	−0.7208	+1.035
		10	Male	30.0 (5.0)	Wing Chun	...	43.4 (4.0)			
Lai et al 1993	Cross-sectional	21	Male	58.7 (3.9)	Tai Chi	Yang, 108 postures	33.9 (6.3)	+1.3836	+0.7252	+2.0421
		23	Male	59.1 (4.0)	Sedentary	...	26.3 (4.4)			
		20	Female	58.3 (4.8)	Tai Chi	Yang, 108 postures	21.8 (2.2)	+0.8943	+0.2834	+1.5052
		26	Female	57.5 (4.7)	Sedentary	...	19.0 (3.6)			
Lan et al 1996	Cross-sectional	22	Male	70.4 (4.1)	Tai Chi	Yang, 108 postures	26.9 (4.7)	+1.2289	+0.5503	+1.9076
		18	Male	69.5 (4.2)	Sedentary	...	21.8 (3.1)			
		19	Female	66.9 (2.7)	Tai Chi	Yang,108 postures	20.1 (2.9)	+1.3965	+0.6670	+2.1260
		17	Female	67.1 (2.8)	Sedentary	...	16.5 (2.0)			

Note: LBCI denotes lower bound confidence interval; UBCI denotes upper bound confidence interval. Effect size is not significant if 0 is included in the confidence interval.
*Matched on gender, age, and body composition.

Copyright © 2006. Lippincott Williams & Wilkins. *Study Guide to Accompany Essentials of Nursing Research*, by Denise F. Polit and Cheryl Tatano Beck.

Effect sizes are important for power calculations when designing research studies and help clinicians and researchers understand the magnitude and direction of a relationship.[33,34]

The following formula[34] was used:

$$ES_{sm} = \frac{Mean_{Rx} - Mean_C}{S_{pool}}$$

Where Rx denotes Tai Chi exercise group, C denotes control or comparison group, and

$$S_{pool} = \sqrt{\frac{(n_1 - 1)s_1^2 + (n_2 - 1)s_2^2}{n_1 + n_2 - 2}}$$

where n = sample size and s = standard deviation.

D-STAT* software was used to calculate the ES_{sm} and the 95% confidence intervals. The ES_{sm} for each study was weighted by the sample size and pooled variance. The postintervention mean aerobic capacity ($\dot{V}o_2$ peak) was used to contrast the experimental and control group in the experimental studies, as there was no difference in the baseline mean scores in these studies. The ES_{sm} for 1 of the experimental studies[20] was calculated by D-STAT using the mean change in aerobic capacity, because of incomplete descriptive data. The ES_{sm} in the cross-sectional studies were derived from group contrasts between the Tai Chi exercise and the comparison groups. All relevant data derived from the studies were coded and entered into SPSS (10.0)[35] for analysis.

INTERPRETATION OF EFFECT SIZES

Cohen[33] has previously presented guidelines for assessing effect sizes. An effect size (ES) of 0.20 is judged to be a small effect, 0.50 as a medium effect, and 0.80 as a large effect.[33] In addition, a proportion of variance (η^2) can be calculated. Analysis of variance is a t-test statistic for means greater than 2. The analysis of variance ES is called f; and $f = d/2$. Using the formula $\eta^2 = [d^2/(d^2 + 4)]$, the percentage of variance between 2 groups can be calculated.[33] Finally, interpretation of the ES can be expanded by transforming the ES into a percentile. The percentile is obtained by referring to a normal distribution table and identifying the area under the curve associated with the ES, referred to as the measure of nonoverlap, (U_3).[33] U_3 is the percentage of the control distribution exceeded by the upper 50% of the treatment population.[36] U_3 readily provides the clinician with information regarding the success or failure of a treatment or intervention. For example, if the ES = 0.85, then 80% of the control group is below the average person in the treatment group. Also, it is important to note that when 50% of the control group is below the average person in the treatment group, then the ES = 0 (eg, no nonoverlap).[32,33,36]

---

*Johnson, BT D-STAT: Software for the Meta-Analytic Review of Research Literature. Lawrence Erlbaum Associates, Inc; 1989.

Copyright © 2006. Lippincott Williams & Wilkins. *Study Guide to Accompany Essentials of Nursing Research*, by Denise F. Polit and Cheryl Tatano Beck.

■ Results

DESCRIPTIVE DATA FROM STUDIES IN META-ANALYSIS

Quality scores ranged from 22 to 28 (mean = 25.1, SD = 2.0) and no studies were excluded on the basis of their quality. The purpose of each study was clearly defined in all of the studies included in the meta-analysis. All but 1 of the studies had a complete and comprehensive description of subject characteristics. All of the studies had the dependent variable (aerobic capacity) clearly defined. However, only 1 of the 7 studies had the rater blinded to group assignment when collecting the data on aerobic capacity.

Within these studies, a total of 344 subjects participated; 166 subjects were in Tai Chi exercise groups. There were 82 males and 57 females, and no gender was specified for the remaining 27 subjects practicing Tai Chi. There were 178 subjects in either control or comparison groups. Sample sizes ranged from 7 to 27 subjects per group. Mainly, healthy older adults participated in these studies (n = 6). In the Tai Chi exercise groups, on average men were 56.0 years old (SD = 12.3) and women were 60.4 years old (SD = 7.0). Control/comparison groups were similar with regard to age and health status (men = 55.5 years, SD = 14.2; women = 60.9 years, SD = 6.4).

Four of the 7 studies had subjects perform the classical Yang style of Tai Chi, which constitutes 108 postures. One study had a modified 13-movement Yang style of Tai Chi, while Tai Chi styles were unspecified in 2 of the studies. In the 2 experimental studies, the duration of the Tai Chi exercise sessions ranged from 45 to 60 minutes, 3 to 5 times per week. The length of the Tai Chi intervention-training period ranged from 12 to 52 weeks. The workload of the outcome variable, aerobic capacity, was provided either by treadmill or cycle ergometer in all of the studies.

In 6 of the studies,[2,4,5,19,25,30] aerobic capacity was derived from $\dot{V}o_2$ peak through estimations obtained from subjects' expired air. One study[20] used predicted maximal workload using published equations by plotting heart rate and estimating workload at the predicted maximal heart rate. Thus $\dot{V}o_2$ max is not likely to have been achieved in these studies. Though use of $\dot{V}o_2$ peak and established equations for estimating oxygen consumption during exercise testing is common, aerobic capacity may have been overestimated due to wide variance inherent with multistage testing.[27,28]

EFFECTS OF TAI CHI ON AEROBIC CAPACITY

The effect size and the 95% confidence interval were calculated for each study, weighted by the sample size and pooled variance. Effects of Tai Chi exercise on aerobic capacity in this meta-analysis also included study design, gender, physical activity habits, style of Tai Chi exercise, and the length of the Tai Chi exercise intervention-training period. The percent of variance between groups (η^2) and the measure of nonoverlap (U_3), was only calculated for effects found to be statistically significant (Table 3).

The average effect size for the cross-sectional studies was large (ES_{sm} = 1.01; CI = +0.37, +1.66) (Fig 1), while in the experimental studies the average effect size was small (ES_{sm} = 0.33; CI = −0.41, +1.07) (Fig 2). In the cross-sectional studies, approximately 20% (η^2 = 0.20) of the variance in aerobic capacity could be explained by

Copyright © 2006. Lippincott Williams & Wilkins. *Study Guide to Accompany Essentials of Nursing Research*, by Denise F. Polit and Cheryl Tatano Beck.

TABLE 3 Aerobic Capacity Effects Sizes and 95% Confidence Intervals ($n = 344$)

Selected Group for Analysis	n	ES	LBCI	UBCI	η^2	U_3
Study Design						
Cross-sectional	186	1.01*	+0.37	+1.66	0.20	0.84
Experimental	158	0.33	−0.41	+1.07		
Gender[†]						
Women	126	0.83	−0.43	+2.09		
Men	167	0.65	−0.04	+1.34		
Physical Activity Level						
Sedentary comparisons	253	0.80*	+0.19	+1.41	0.14	0.79
Other exercise	91	0.22	−0.81	+1.24		
Style of Tai Chi						
Classical Yang style	224	1.10*	+0.82	+1.38	0.23	0.86
Modified or unspecified	120	−0.17	−0.54	+0.20		
Length of Tai Chi Intervention[‡]						
52 weeks	58	0.94*	+0.06	+1.81	0.18	0.83
12 or 16 weeks[§]	100	−0.28*	−0.53	−0.02	0.02	0.61

Note: n denotes sample size; ES, effect size; LBCI, lower bound confidence interval; UBCI, upper bound confidence interval; η^2 = percent of explained variance between groups (η^2) and U_3 = percentage of the treatment group above the control group mean. The effect size is not significant if 0 is included in the confidence interval; η^2 and U_3 are reported only for significant ES.
*significant ES.
[†]51 subjects not included due incomplete descriptive data.
[‡] Sample of 158 subjects.
[§]Control group better than 61% of the subjects in treatment group.

group. Aerobic capacity for the average subject in a Tai Chi exercise group was higher than 84% of the subjects in the comparison groups in the cross-sectional studies.

Six of the 7 studies[2,4,5,19,25,30] reported gender-specific descriptive statistics and enabled gender-specific effects to be calculated. Effect sizes of aerobic capacity in women ($ES_{sm} = 0.83$; CI = −0.43, +2.09) were somewhat higher than those for men ($ES_{sm} = 0.65$; CI = −0.04, +1.34), though not statistically significant.

Effect sizes examining aerobic capacity based on the physical activity habits of subjects in the control and comparison groups were also calculated. Four of the studies[4,5,19,30] had sedentary subjects as comparisons, while the other 3 studies[2,20,25] involved subjects doing other exercise, such as walking. Approximately 14% ($\eta^2 = 0.14$) of the variance in aerobic capacity could be explained by physical activity habits. Aerobic capacity for the subjects in a Tai Chi exercise group was higher than 79% of the sedentary subjects (average $ES_{sm} = 0.80$; CI = +0.19, +1.41).

Dose-treatment effects of Tai Chi exercise were calculated by the style of Tai Chi exercise performed. Four of the 7 studies[2,4,5,30] utilized the longest form of the Yang style of Tai Chi with 108 postures. The other 3 studies had subjects perform a simplified Yang style form (13 movements)[20] or the style of Tai Chi was not specified in 2 of the studies.[19,25] Approximately 23% ($\eta^2 = 0.23$) of the variance in aerobic capacity could be explained by style of Tai Chi exercise. Aerobic capacity for the average subject performing

Copyright © 2006. Lippincott Williams & Wilkins. *Study Guide to Accompany Essentials of Nursing Research*, by Denise F. Polit and Cheryl Tatano Beck.

Tai Chi & Aerobic Capacity ES (95% C.I.)

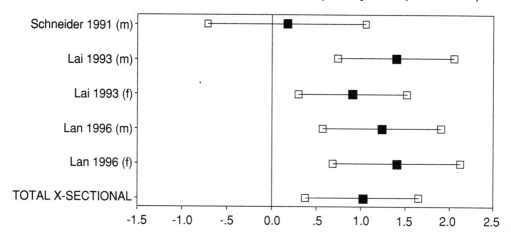

ES=effect size, C.I.=confidence interval, m=males, f=females

All studies listed by 1st Author and year; ES not significant if 0 in CI

FIGURE 1. Cross-sectional studies, $n = 3$.

Tai Chi & Aerobic Capacity ES (95% C.I.)

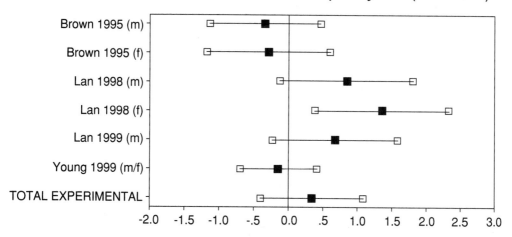

ES=effect size, C.I.=confidence interval, m=males, f=females

All studies listed by 1st Author and year; ES not significant if 0 in CI

FIGURE 2. Experimental studies, $n = 4$.

Copyright © 2006. Lippincott Williams & Wilkins. *Study Guide to Accompany Essentials of Nursing Research*, by Denise F. Polit and Cheryl Tatano Beck.

the classical Yang style form of Tai Chi exercise was higher than 86% of the subjects in the control or comparison groups (average $ES_{sm} = 1.10$; CI $= +0.82, +1.38$).

In the 4 experimental studies,[2,4,19,20] Tai Chi exercise session ranged from 45 to 60 minutes (mean $= 56$ minutes, SD $= 7.5$), 3 to 5 times per week (mean $= 4$ times per week, SD $= 0.8$). The length of Tai Chi intervention training period ranged from 12 to 52 weeks (mean $= 33$ weeks, SD $= 22$). Only effect sizes examining aerobic capacity based on length of the Tai Chi intervention were calculated. Approximately 18% ($\eta^2 = 0.18$) of the variance in aerobic capacity could be explained by length of the Tai Chi exercise-training period. Aerobic capacity for the average subject participating in a 52-week Tai Chi exercise group was higher than 83% of the subjects in the control group (average $ES_{sm} = 0.94$; CI $= +0.06, +1.18$). On the other hand, the improvement in aerobic capacity for the average subject in the 12-week or 16-week control group was better than 61% of the subjects in the Tai Chi exercise group (average $ES_{sm} = -0.28$, CI $= -0.53, -0.02$). However, this result is not likely to be clinically relevant, only 2% ($\eta^2 = 0.02$) of the variance in aerobic capacity could be explained by the number of weeks subjects remained in the control condition.

■ Discussion

Given the limited number of studies pertaining to the effects of Tai Chi exercise on aerobic capacity in women ($n = 126$), these results need to be interpreted with caution. However, this early review appears to indicate potential gender differences in the effectiveness of Tai Chi exercise on aerobic capacity. Effect sizes of Tai Chi exercise on aerobic capacity in women were greater than those for men, though not statistically significant. This finding suggests that it may be important to consider, and future studies could clarify if there are gender differences by designing stratified randomization (based on gender). The development of alternative exercise programs for women including Tai Chi exercise could be of value, as previous research has reported that women desired exercise options other than using the treadmill or cycle.[37] Further, 1 of the experimental studies[20] did not provide gender information for the subjects completing the study. It is unknown if an effect based on gender would have resulted in different findings.

The degree of improvement in aerobic capacity depends on the exercise intensity, duration, and frequency, as well as the subject's initial level of physical activity. Persons who were sedentary before beginning Tai Chi exercise made greater gains with a more favorable effect. This finding is consistent with the traditional western exercise literature wherein the most sedentary persons demonstrate the greatest benefit when they initiate a regular program of exercise.[38] However, consideration needs to be given to possible selection bias, as Tai Chi masters were compared with sedentary subjects (>5 years), matched on age and gender, in 2 of the cross-sectional studies.[5,30] This selection of subjects with distinctly different exercise proficiencies is likely to influence the large effect sizes obtained. Further, the extent to which diet and other lifestyle practices influenced the results was not measured.

Tai Chi exercise styles varied among the studies reviewed. The classical Yang style comprises 108 postures and is more difficult to learn.[5,30] Simpler forms have fewer

Copyright © 2006. Lippincott Williams & Wilkins. *Study Guide to Accompany Essentials of Nursing Research*, by Denise F. Polit and Cheryl Tatano Beck.

postures and exclude some of the more strenuous movements, such as deep squatting or vigorous kicking. While the simplified forms of Tai Chi are shorter and easier to learn, they may have a reduced training benefit. The 4 studies[2,4,5,30] that utilized the classical Yang style of Tai Chi had larger effect sizes. The findings are likely due to the inclusion of more strenuous movements and the longer time needed to complete the entire set of postures.

In the 4 experimental studies, the Tai Chi exercise intervention ranged from 45 to 60 minutes, 3 to 5 times per week, and is consistent with the current recommendations for western-style exercise.[27,28] However, the length of the Tai Chi intervention training period varied, ranging from 12 to 52 weeks. Subjects in 2 of the 4 experimental studies[2,4] had longer intervention times (52 weeks) than the other 2 experimental studies (12 or 16 weeks).[19,20] The largest effect was seen in the studies with the 52-week intervention time. However, the improvement in aerobic capacity for the average subject in the 12-week or 16-week control group was significantly better than subjects in the Tai Chi exercise groups. This finding may partially be attributed to a threshold effect when performing Tai Chi exercise or a dropout effect.

Subjects in the 12-week or 16-week Tai Chi exercise groups participated in either a simplified or unspecified form of Tai Chi and may have had a reduced training benefit. In the study by Young and colleagues,[20] moderate-intensity aerobic exercise, instead of sedentary controls, may partially explain why the improvement in aerobic capacity for the average 12-week control subject was greater than the average subject in the Tai Chi exercise group. Further, the mean change in aerobic capacity within and between the 12-week or 16-week control and Tai Chi exercise groups was small in these 2 studies.

Finally, the dropout rate for subjects participating in a 52-week intervention was approximately 26.5%, while the 12-week and 16-week intervention studies reported dropout rates of 17% and 8% respectively. Future research could help explain these findings by examining dose-response effects of Tai Chi exercise.

■ Conclusion

The findings of this meta-analysis fill a gap in the literature and highlight a potential benefit in aerobic capacity when performing Tai Chi. This meta-analysis included a total of 7 studies, only 4 of which used an experimental design. It is likely that the small samples in these studies had insufficient power for the researchers to detect significant differences between groups, assuming that $\alpha = .05$ and power $= 0.80$ were utilized.

Tai Chi may be an additional form of aerobic exercise, suitable for sedentary older adults and those with heart disease.[2,3,20] The slow and graceful movements of Tai Chi have several advantages over other forms of exercise, as Tai Chi does not require any special clothing or equipment, making Tai Chi a cost-effective and affordable form of exercise. Tai Chi may also foster adherence due to its practical utility (may be performed any time and at any place). Moreover, Tai Chi might be an enjoyable and preferred form of exercise for some.[1]

Future research studies examining the effect the Tai Chi on aerobic capacity should consider using the same frequency, duration, and intensity of Tai Chi exercise as that

Copyright © 2006. Lippincott Williams & Wilkins. *Study Guide to Accompany Essentials of Nursing Research*, by Denise F. Polit and Cheryl Tatano Beck.

recommended by the American College of Sports Medicine.[27,28] This is necessary in order to have valid comparisons of the effect of Tai Chi exercise to traditional forms of exercise, such as walking. Further, it is recommended that an established style of Tai Chi be used, such as the classical Yang style, rather than unspecified or modified forms, so as to provide a comparison to published findings. Research among diverse populations, including persons with chronic diseases, would help to expand current knowledge about the effect of Tai Chi on aerobic capacity. However, aerobic capacity is only 1 potential outcome, and improvements in balance,[7–9] muscular strength,[10–12] flexibility,[5,13,14] relaxation[15,16] and mood state[15,17–19] may be additional benefits of doing Tai Chi.

Ruth E. Taylor-Piliae, RN, CNS, MN
Doctoral Candidate, Department of Physiological Nursing, School of Nursing, University of California, San Francisco, Calif.
Erika S. Froelicher, RN, MPH, PhD, FAAN
Professor, Department of Physiological Nursing, School of Nursing, University of California, San Francisco; Calif.
This research project was supported by grant 1 F31 NR08180-01 from the National Center for Complementary and Alternative Medicine and the National Institutes of Health, US Department of Health and Human Services and a Graduate Opportunity Fellowship from the University of California, San Francisco, awarded to Ruth Taylor-Piliae.
The authors thank Dr Kathryn A. Lee for her advice and helpful comments on previous drafts of this article and Dr Steven M. Paul for his assistance with the statistical analyses.
Corresponding author
Ruth E. Taylor-Piliae, RN, CNS, MN, Department of Physiological Nursing, School of Nursing, 2 Koret Way, Box 0610, San Francisco, CA 94143 (e-mail: rtaylor@itsa.uscf.edu).

REFERENCES

1. Kutner NG, Barnhart H, Wolf SL, McNeely E, Xu T. Self-report benefits of Tai Chi practice by older adults. *J Gerontol B Psychol Sci Soc Sci. 1997; 52:*P242–P246.
2. Lan C, Chen SY, Lai JS, Wong MK. The effect of Tai Chi on cardiorespiratory function in patients with coronary artery bypass surgery. *Med Sci Sports Exerc.* 1999;31:634–638.
3. Channer KS, Barrow D, Barrow R, Osborne M, Ives G. Changes in haemodynamic parameters following Tai Chi Chuan and aerobic exercise in patients recovering from acute myocardial infarction. *Postgrad Med J.* 1996;72:349–351.
4. Lan C, Lai JS, Chen SY, Wong MK. 12-month Tai Chi training in the elderly: its effect on health fitness. *Med Sci Sports Exerc.* 1998;30:345–351.
5. Lan C, Lai JS, Wong MK, Yu ML. Cardiorespiratory function, flexibility, and body composition among geriatric Tai Chi Chuan practitioners. *Arch Phys Med Rehabil.* 1996;77:612–616.
6. Lai JS, Lan C, Wong MK, Teng SH. Two-year trends in cardiorespiratory function among older Tai Chi Chuan practitioners and sedentary subjects. *J Am Geriatr Soc.* 1995;43:1222–1227.
7. Wolf SL, Coogler C, Xu T. Exploring the basis for Tai Chi Chuan as a therapeutic exercise approach. *Arch Phys Med Rehabil.* 1997;78:886–892.
8. Yan JH. Tai Chi practice improves senior citizens' balance and arm movement control. *J Aging Phys Activity.* 1998;6:271–284.
9. Hain TC, Fuller L, Weil L, Kotsias J. Effects of T'ai Chi on balance. *Arch Otolaryngol Head Neck Surg.* 1999;125:1191–1195.
10. Parker MG, Hocking K, Katus J, Stockert E, Gruby R. The effects of a three-week Tai Chi exercise program on isometric muscle strength and balance in community-dwelling older adults: a pilot study. *Issues Aging.* 2000;23:9–13.
11. Wolfson L, Whipple R, Derby C, et al. Balance and strength training in older adults: intervention gains and Tai Chi maintenance. *J Am Geriat Soc.* 1996;44:498–506.

Copyright © 2006. Lippincott Williams & Wilkins. *Study Guide to Accompany Essentials of Nursing Research*, by Denise F. Polit and Cheryl Tatano Beck.

12. Lan C, Lai JS, Chen SY, Wong MK. Tai Chi Chuan to improve muscular strength and endurance in elderly individuals: a pilot study. *Arch Phys Med Rehabil.* 2000;81:604–607.
13. Hugel K, Sciandra T. The effects of a 12-week Tai Chi program on thoracolumbar, hip and knee flexion in adults 50 years and older. *Issues Aging.* 2000;23:15–18.
14. Hong Y, Li JX, Robinson PD. Balance control, flexibility, and cardiorespiratory fitness among older Tai Chi practitioners. *Br J Sports Med.* 2000;34:29–34.
15. Jin P. Efficacy of Tai Chi, brisk walking, meditation, and reading in reducing mental and emotional stress. *J Psychosom Res.* 1992;36:361–370.
16. Sun WY, Dosch M, Gilmore GD, Pemberton W, Scarseth T. Effects of a Tai Chi Chuan program on Hmong American older adults. *Educ Gerontol.* 1996;22:161–167.
17. Ross MC, Bohannon AS, Davis DC, Gurchiek L. The effects of a short-term exercise program on movement, pain, and mood in the elderly. Results of a pilot study. *J Holist Nurs.* 1999;17:139–147.
18. Jin P. Changes in heart rate, noradrenaline, cortisol and mood during Tai Chi. *J Psychosom Res.* 1989;33:197–206.
19. Brown DR, Wang Y, Ward A, et al. Chronic psychological effects of exercise and exercise plus cognitive strategies. *Med Sci Sports Exerc.* 1995;27:765–775.
20. Young DR, Appel LJ, Jee S, Miller ER III. The effects of aerobic exercise and T'ai Chi on blood pressure in older people: results of a randomized trial. *J Am Geriatr Soc.* 1999;47:277–284.
21. Taylor-Piliae RE. Tai Chi as an adjunct to cardiac rehabilitation exercise training. *J Cardiopulm Rehabil.* 2003;23:90–96.
22. Lan C, Chen SY, Lai JS, Wong MK. Heart rate responses and oxygen consumption during Tai Chi Chuan practice. *Am J Chin Med.* 2001;29:403–410.
23. Lan C, Lai JS, Chen SY. Tai Chi Chuan: an ancient wisdom on exercise and health promotion. *Sports Med.* 2002;32:217–224.
24. Zhuo D, Shephard RJ, Plyley MJ, Davis GM. Cardiorespiratory and metabolic responses during Tai Chi Chuan exercise. *Can J Appl Sport Sci.* 1984;9:7–10.
25. Schneider D, Leung R. Metabolic and cardiorespiratory responses to the performance of Wing Chun and T'ai Chi Chuan exercise. *Int J Sports Med.* 1991;12:319–323.
26. Fontana JA. The energy costs of a modified form of T'ai Chi exercise. *Nurs Res.* 2000;49:91–96.
27. American College of Sports Medicine (ACSM). *ACSM's Resource Manual for Guidelines for Prescription Testing and Prescription.* Philadelphia: Lippincott Williams & Wilkins; 2001.
28. American College of Sports Medicine (ACSM). *ACSM's Guidelines for Exercise Testing and Prescription.* Philadelphia: Lippincott Williams & Wilkins; 2000.
29. Fletcher GF, Balady GJ, Amsterdam EA, et al. Exercise standards for testing and training: a statement for healthcare professionals from the American Heart Association. *Circulation.* 2001;104:1694–1740.
30. Lai JS, Wong MK, Lan C, Chong CK, Lien IN. Cardiorespiratory responses of Tai Chi Chuan practitioners and sedentary subjects during cycle ergometry. *J Formos Med Assoc.* 1993;92:894–899.
31. Chan WW, Bartlett DJ. Effectiveness of Tai Chi as therapeutic exercise in improving balance and postural control. *Phys Occup Ther Geriatr.* 2000;17:1–22.
32. Lee KA. Meta-analysis: a third alternative for student research experience. *Nurse Educ.* 1988;13:30–33.
33. Cohen J. *Statistical Power Analysis for the Behavioral Sciences.* Hillsdale, NJ: Lawerence Erlbaum; 1988.
34. Lipsey MW, Wilson DB. *Practical Meta-Analysis.* Thousand Oaks, Calif: Sage; 2001.
35. Norusis MJ. *SPSS 10.0: Guide to Data Analysis.* Upper Saddle River, NJ: Prentice-Hall; 2000.
36. Lipsey MW. *Design Sensitivity: Statistical Power for Experimental Research.* Newbury Park, Calif: Sage; 1990.
37. Moore SM. Women's views of cardiac rehabilitation programs. *J Cardiopulm Rehabil.* 1996;16:123–129.
38. Haskell WL. JB Wolffe Memorial Lecture. Health consequences of physical activity: understanding and challenges regarding dose-response. *Med Sci Sports Exerc.* 1994;26:649–660.

Copyright © 2006. Lippincott Williams & Wilkins. *Study Guide to Accompany Essentials of Nursing Research,* by Denise F. Polit and Cheryl Tatano Beck.

MOTHERING MULTIPLES

A META-SYNTHESIS OF QUALITATIVE RESEARCH

Cheryl Tatano Beck, DNSc, CNM, FAAN

Increasing numbers of qualitative studies in maternal-child nursing are being published. However, clinical application and knowledge development based on those
studies will be hampered unless the rich understandings gleaned from these individual studies can be synthesized. Meta-synthesis is one technique to help accumulate
knowledge from qualitative research. The first section of this article explains the technique of meta-synthesis and reviews meta-syntheses published in nursing. The focus
then becomes an illustration of a meta-synthesis in maternal-child nursing: Mothering multiples during the first year of life. Six qualitative studies comprised the sample
for the meta-synthesis. The meta-synthesis revealed a shared set of five themes that
help increase our understanding of mothering multiples: "bearing the burden," "rid-
ing an emotional roller coaster," "lifesaving support," "striving for maternal justice,"
and "acknowledging individuality." Implications for practice derived from this meta-
synthesis are addressed.

■ **Key Words:** *Meta-synthesis; Multiple births*

Over the past decade the number of qualitative research studies conducted in maternal-
child nursing has risen substantially, and has spanned the spectrum of maternal-child
nursing from women's pregnancy experiences in prison (Wismont, 2000) to postpartum
depressed mothers' experiences interacting with their children (Beck, 1996) to stressful
life experiences in 9- to 11-year-old children (Jacobson, 1994).

Although qualitative studies in maternal-child nursing are increasing, their clinical
application and their contribution to knowledge development will be impeded unless
the rich understandings gleaned from these individual studies can be synthesized.
Meta-synthesis is an approach that can be used in this regard. The focus of this article is
on describing the results of a meta-synthesis of qualitative studies that have explored the
experience of mothering multiples during the first year of life.

Reprinted with permission from *MCN* 2002; 27 [4]: 214–221.

Copyright © 2006. Lippincott Williams & Wilkins. *Study Guide to Accompany Essentials
of Nursing Research*, by Denise F. Polit and Cheryl Tatano Beck.

■ What is Meta-Synthesis?

Schreiber, Crooks, and Stern (1997) define meta-synthesis as "the aggregating of a group of studies for the purpose of discovering the essential elements and translating the results into the end product that transforms the original results into a new conceptualization" (p. 314). Meta-synthesis helps us accumulate knowledge from individual studies, thus assisting us to utilize the information learned from the studies clinically. Meta-synthesis is a rigorous scientific technique. Sandelowski and colleagues (1997) warn that synthesizing qualitative research involves "carefully peeling away the surface layers of studies to find their hearts and souls in a way that does the least damage to them" (p. 370). Researchers conducting a meta-synthesis walk a fine line between needing to analyze the studies in enough detail to maintain the integrity of each specific study, while trying to avoid becoming so immersed in the details that the synthesis is unusable (Sandelowski, 1997).

Debate surrounds the issue of synthesizing studies using different qualitative approaches, such as synthesizing phenomenology and grounded theory in one meta-synthesis. Some believe that different qualitative approaches should not be mixed together because of their differing philosophical underpinnings. However, others are less concerned about differing qualitative methods and are more concerned with focusing on the same substantive area (Schreiber et al., 1997).

■ A Review of Selected Published Meta-Syntheses in Nursing

Four meta-syntheses in the nursing literature are reviewed here. These qualitative syntheses focused on wellness-illness, threats to the integrity of self, courage among persons experiencing lingering threats to their well being, and living with HIV infection.

Jensen and Allen (1994) conducted syntheses of 112 qualitative studies on the *individual's experience of wellness and illness* from 1980 to 1991. Studies reporting the use of qualitative designs regarding health, disease, wellness, and illness in adults were part of the inclusion criteria. Twenty-seven of these studies used a grounded theory approach and were synthesized together to describe the process inherent in living with health and disease. The authors labeled this process "work-of-living" with health disease and it consisted of five phases:

1. recognizing the threat,
2. defending and protecting self,
3. reconciling the change,
4. learning to live again, and
5. living again.

Jensen and Allen then synthesized 35 phenomenologic studies to describe the experience of health and disease. Synthesis of these studies revealed that the lived experience of health-disease was "one of abiding vitality, transitional harmony, rhythmical connectedness, unfolding fulfillment, active optimism, and reflective transformation" (p. 354). The

Copyright © 2006. Lippincott Williams & Wilkins. *Study Guide to Accompany Essentials of Nursing Research*, by Denise F. Polit and Cheryl Tatano Beck.

synthesis of the 50 remaining studies, which included ethnographic studies and descriptive/exploratory studies, revealed that the context of health-disease is one of body, space, time, and human relationships of being-in-the-world of health-disease.

Morse's (1997) meta-synthesis of qualitative studies that examined *responses to a threat to the integrity of the self* revealed a five-stage theory. Stage 1, *Vigilance*, includes responses of suspecting, reading the body, observing, becoming overwhelmed, maintaining emotional control, and accepting assistance. Stage 2, *Disruption: Enduring To Survive*, consists of holding on, being in shattered reality, and experiencing a "haze of disorientation." In Stage 3, *Enduring To Live: Striving To Regain Self*, the responses utilized were living through the pain, trying to bear it, accepting dependence, recognizing physical change and loss of function, fearing isolation, grasping the implications of illness/injury, and recognizing the uncertain prognosis. Stage 4, *Suffering: Striving to Restore Self*, includes struggling with grief, doing the work of healing, and making sense. Stage 5, *Learning to Live With the Altered Self*, is the final phase. Responses involved are getting to know and trust the altered body, accepting the consequences of the experience, revaluing the experience, obtaining mastery, and revising life goals.

Courage among persons who were experiencing a variety of lingering threats to their well-being was the focus of Finfgeld's (1999) meta-synthesis. She synthesized six qualitative studies and reported that courage is a dynamic phenomenon that is intiated by a perceived threat. Courage was envisioned as a process of efforts to fully accept reality, problem solve, and push beyond the struggles. Thriving and personal integrity are two outcomes of being courageous. Both intrapersonal and interpersonal factors are needed to help maintain courage.

A meta-synthesis of 21 qualitative research studies on living with HIV infection was conducted by Barroso and Powell-Cope (2000). Six overarching metaphors emerged that described the experience of adults living with HIV infection. These metaphors entailed finding meaning in the disease, shattered meaning, human connectedness, focus on self, negotiating healthcare, and dealing with stigma.

▪ How to Conduct a Meta-Synthesis

Noblit and Hare (1988) proposed the following seven phases that comprise the conduct of a meta-synthesis:

Phase 1: Getting started. In this first step the researcher identifies an area of interest that qualitative studies might inform.

Phase 2: Deciding what is relevant to the initial interest. The researcher must decide which qualitative studies are relevant for the meta-synthesis.

Phase 3: Reading the studies. The researcher reads and rereads the qualitative studies to identify the key metaphors, themes, or concepts.

Phase 4: Determining how the studies are related. In conducting a meta-synthesis, the researcher needs to "put together" the specific studies in the sample by deciding how the studies are related (Nobit & Hare, 1988, p. 28). Helpful in this step is creating a list and comparing key themes, metaphors, or concepts for each qualitative study. Studies can be related in three ways: reciprocal (directly comparable), refutational (in opposition to each

Copyright © 2006. Lippincott Williams & Wilkins. *Study Guide to Accompany Essentials of Nursing Research*, by Denise F. Polit and Cheryl Tatano Beck.

other), and in line of agreement (studies grounded together represent a line of argument instead of being reciprocal or refutational).

Phase 5: Translating the studies into one another. Metaphors or themes in one study are compared with those in other studies. An adequate translation is one that keeps the key metaphors or themes of each study in their relation to other metaphors or concepts in the same study and also with other studies in the meta-synthesis (Noblit & Hare, 1988).

Phase 6: Synthesizing translations. After translating studies into one another, the next challenge for the researcher is to make a whole into more than the individual parts imply.

Phase 7: Expressing the synthesis. In this final step, the results of the meta-synthesis are documented and reported.

■ A Meta-Synthesis of Qualitative Research on Mothering Multiples

A review of the literature using databases such as *CINAHL, Psylit,* and *Medline* revealed six qualitative studies on mothering multiples during the first year of life. Characteristics of these studies, published over a 19-year period between 1980 and 1999, are located in Table 1. The earliest study, published in 1980, investigated the mothering of twins, triplets, and quadruplets (Goshen-Gottstein, 1980). Robin, Josse, and Tourrette (1988) focused their study on early mother-twin interaction. The one grounded theory study included in this meta-synthesis was conducted by Anderson and Anderson (1990). Their substantive theory described how mothers developed a relationship with twins during their first year of life. The fourth study included in the meta-synthesis examined maternal reactions to the birth of triplets (Robin, Bydlowski, Cahen, & Josse, 1991). Garel and Blondel (1992) also focused their research on mothers of triplets. These two authors assessed the psychological consequences of having triplets (at 1 year of age). Holditch-Davis, Roberts, and Sandelowski (1999) published the most recent study in this meta-synthesis. Couples' perception of parenting multiple birth infants was the focus of this qualitative portion of their study.

These six qualitative studies were synthesized using Noblit and Hare's (1998) seven-stage method. For each of the studies a list of their key metaphors/themes was made and then these lists were juxtaposed (Table 2). The content in Table 2 is directly derived from the studies and had not yet been translated. After reviewing each study in depth, a decision was made that all the studies were directly comparable as reciprocal translations. As other nursing analysts have done, this author went beyond Noblit and Hare's approach in Phase 6 to create a unified description of the phenomenon under study which pooled all six studies. The meta-synthesis revealed a shared set of five themes that increase the understanding of the experience of mothering multiples during the first year after delivery:

1. BEARING THE BURDEN

Mothers of multiples bear the heavy burden of child care 24 hours a day, 7 days a week. These women are on maternal task overload with their physical and mental reserves being severely stretched and grossly overtaxed. For mothers of multiples there is no

Copyright © 2006. Lippincott Williams & Wilkins. *Study Guide to Accompany Essentials of Nursing Research,* by Denise F. Polit and Cheryl Tatano Beck.

TABLE 1 Set of Studies Included in Mothering Multiples Meta-Synthesis

Author(s)/Year	Country	Sample	Research Design	Data Collection	Data Collection Times (Infant's Age)
Goshen-Gottstein (1980)	Israel	4 mothers of twins, 6 mothers of triplets, 4 mothers of quadruplets	Descriptive, Qualitative*	Observation/Interviews	Birth to 4–6 yrs
Robin, Josse, & Tourrette (1988)	France	1) 7 mothers of twins, 2) 21 mothers of twins	Descriptive, Qualitative	Observation/Interviews	1) Birth to 3 yrs 2) 1 yr
Anderson & Anderson (1990)	Canada	10 mothers of twins	Grounded theory	Interviews	1 mo to 1 yr
Robin, Bydlowski, Cahen, & Josse (1991)	France	14 mothers of triplets	Descriptive, Qualitative	Observation/Interviews	4 mos to 1 yr
Garel & Blondel (1992)	France	12 mothers of triplets	Descriptive, Qualitative	Interviews	1 yr
Holditch-Davis, Roberts, & Sandelowski (1999)	United States	Sets of mothers and fathers: 7 of twins, 1 of triplets	Descriptive, Qualitative	Observation/Interviews	1 wk to 3 mos

*This term was given to a qualitative study that used a theory-generating paradigm but did not identify a specific qualitative design such as phenomenology or grounded theory

Copyright © 2006. Lippincott Williams & Wilkins. *Study Guide to Accompany Essentials of Nursing Research*, by Denise F. Polit and Cheryl Tatano Beck.

TABLE 2 Metaphors Used to Construct Reciprocal Translations in Mothering Multiples Meta-Synthesis

Themes	Goshen-Gottstein (1980)	Robin et al. (1988)	Anderson & Anderson (1990, 1991)	Robin et al. (1992)	Garel & Blondel (1999)	Holditch-Davis et al.
Myriad of Emotions	Mothers' ambivalence	—	—	General emotional conditions: • feelings of abnormality, • predominance of depressive reactions • defensive reactions • feelings of persecution	• Social isolation • Mothers' emotional well-being	—
Practical Burden	Dealing with unusual demands	Overload of baby care	—	Mother-infant: exchanges during child care • emphasis on organization • utilitarian care • no pleasure in interactions	Practical problems	Difficulties in management of multiples
Equality	Treating children equally as a unit, talking to or about children as a unit	1) Be sure to merge twins into a single unit 2) need for equalitarianism	Maternal justice			
Problems of Differentiation	Difficulty of relating to more than 1 or 2 children	• Problems of differentiation • Problems of preference	—	Degree of involvement with triplets • inability to describe triplets reaction	—	Attachment issues with multiples
Individualization	Treating children as individuals	Need for early individualization/ desire for 2 dyadic relationships	• Individualization • Differentiation • Polarization	Predominance of individualized care • ability to describe each triplet • pleasure in interactions	Specificity of mother-child relationships	Specialness of multiples
Coping/Adaptation	Mothers who coped better	Maternal adaptation to triadic situation, father's role	Support	• Feelings of solidarity with other females • Adjustments • Support from father and relatives	• Home help • Marital difficulties	—

Copyright © 2006. Lippincott Williams & Wilkins. *Study Guide to Accompany Essentials of Nursing Research*, by Denise F. Polit and Cheryl Tatano Beck.

down time because caring for more than one infant eliminates any extra time. As one mother shared, "*When you have one and there are two parents, you're off at least half the time but with more than one you can never be off really*" (Holditch-Davis et al., 1999, p. 206).

For a majority of women, mothering their multiple infants results in considerable stress and fatigue. One mother of triplets in Garel and Blondel's (1992) study revealed, "*With three toddlers you constantly have to choose between what you have to do, with what you want to do and what you can do. Sometimes I cant't cope, I give up, I just deal with the most urgent things*" (p. 729). Moments of pleasure, fun, and play with their infants are few and far between because mothers had no time for these "*extras*" (Robin et al., 1988).

Goshen-Gottstein (1980) reported that in her study of mothers of twins, triplets, and quadruplets the central problem for these women was how to care for several infants who all need their attention simultaneously. Mothers often felt guilty making their infants "*wait in line*" (Holditch-Davis et al., 1999, p. 206) to feed. Mothers had to eventually find a "*system*" to juggle care. Each physical task that a mother was able to independently perform was considered a "*real milestone*" in her development as a mother of multiples. In addition to chronic fatigue, the enormity of the child care burden resulted in other physical problems including back pain.

Mothers of multiple infants felt confined and tied down. Women felt they could not even just "*run to the grocery store*" for milk because of the enormity of preparation it required to take more than one infant out of the home (Holditch-Davis et al., 1999, p. 206).

Some mothers of multiples also bore the burden of financial problems due to the birth of their multiple infants (Robin et al., 1991). Their finances were overtaxed by mothers having to stop work and the necessity of moving to a bigger home to accommodate their expanded family.

2. RIDING THE EMOTIONAL ROLLER COASTER

Mothers experience a myriad of emotions over the first year of their multiple infants' lives. These emotions can fluxuate from wonder and gratitude to depression and despair. Mothers in the Holditch-Davis et al. (1999) study remarked on the positive uniqueness of multiple infants. One mother shared that she and her husband "*held them in their arms and stared at them in disbelief and wonder and gratitude at everything*" (p. 206).

A mother of quadruplets described having multiples as "*a blessing, such a blessing that we do not know what to do with it. It is like giving someone a royal meal when be does not know how to eat it*" (Goshen-Gottstein, 1980, p. 193). Other women in the same study described having supertwins as a "*curse.*"

Fulfillment is another positive emotion involved with mothering multiples. "*We wanted a large family. We got it right. When I watch them playing and dancing around, they look so cute! We want to keep them!*" (Garel & Blondel, 1992, p. 731).

Garel and Blondel (1992) studied the psychological consequences of 12 mothers 1 year after giving birth to triplets. One year after a triplet delivery, the majority of women were still experiencing serious psychological troubles. Three mothers were being treated for major depression. The following quote illustrates this emotion: "*I was so depressed*

Copyright © 2006. Lippincott Williams & Wilkins. *Study Guide to Accompany Essentials of Nursing Research*, by Denise F. Polit and Cheryl Tatano Beck.

and completely down-hearted, I was afraid of being alone with the children. Then I became anxious about being a threat to my own life. I had never felt like that before, it was awful" (Garel & Blondel, p. 730).

Six other women in Garel and Blondel's (1992) study experienced serious psychological problems such as anxiety, tension, irritability, and helplessness as noted by one woman's comments: *"When the children started to move around, it was exhausting. Not only physically, it was also a stress. I find it harder now. When they were babies in their cribs I was in control, now I am so nervous, it is a disaster. You lose your mind. With triplets, you need to be well balanced. Sometimes I feel suffocated. I am so tense, trying to get a hold on myself"* (Garel & Blondel, p. 730).

Guilt and frustration are other emotions on this roller coaster. Being unable to enjoy their desired infants resulted in these feelings. *"You cannot really enjoy one child, you always keep in mind the two others waiting for you. It is really frustrating"* (Garel & Blondel, 1992, p. 730).

In Robin et al.'s (1991) study of 14 women's reactions to triplets, 40% of these mothers were depressed, discouraged, and bitter. For some of these mothers, the depression was accompanied by resignation, fatalism, and feelings of being punished.

3. LIFESAVING SUPPORT

Due to the obvious strain on the mothers in caring for their multiple infants, obtaining instrumental and emotional support was crucial. The major source of support for the mother was the multiples' father. In Anderson and Anderson's (1990) study, two types of parenting styles of the fathers were noted. The first type was cooperative parenting where the father did not have to be asked by the mother to help with the child care. Mothers felt confident in these fathers' abilities. One woman described her cooperative husband: *"He does everything except breast-feed them. When he is not working, he contributes at least 50% of their care"* (p. 375). Another mother expressed that her spouse does *"virtually everything for them that a mother would. They respond to him just as easily or as much as they respond to me"* (p. 376). In the second type, assisted parenting, the mothers implemented and orchestrated child care. The fathers participated when problems abounded. These women were mainly responsible for child care and running the household.

In Anderson and Anderson's (1990) study some women perceived their husbands as also providing emotional support. For other women, however, they felt their close girlfriends were better suited to give emotional support. One mother shared that her girlfriend was *"a kindred spirit, a person I can have marathon talk sessions with, one who listens and is accessible, and who knows my playful side as well as my more serious side"* (Anderson & Anderson, p. 376).

Robin and associates (1988) reported in their twin study that in some cases the father assumed a *"surrogate mother"* (p. 157) role. Both the mother and father in tandem undertook child care.

In studying maternal reactions to the birth of triplets, Robin and colleagues (1991) found that help from relatives, especially the father and the grandparents, was a source of moral support, which the mothers desperately needed. For some fathers, the multiple

Copyright © 2006. Lippincott Williams & Wilkins. *Study Guide to Accompany Essentials of Nursing Research,* by Denise F. Polit and Cheryl Tatano Beck.

birth allowed them to more easily assume their paternal roles than had a single infant been born. Other husbands failed to provide their wives with this crucial support due to the inability of these men to accept the multiple births.

The birth of triplets at times frightened family and friends away, leaving the mother isolated and without help (Robin et al., 1991). Mothers in the Robin et al. study described that help from family and friends increased by the triplets fourth month of life. The mothers perceived that by 4 months their family and friends had time to respond to the shock of the multiple births and could better offer help. Mothers of triplets in Garel and Blondel's (1992) study found the opposite pattern of support. As the 1-year mark approached, family, friends, and fathers stopped helping the mothers on a regular basis. The women complained that outside cooperation faded with time and that no one really understood the heavy burden still being carried. As one mother expressed: "*Unless you spend all your days and nights with them, you cannot realize. No words could describe the way things go*" (Garel & Blondel, p. 730).

Multiples support groups were mentioned by mothers in two studies as another lifeline of support (Holditch-Davis et al., 1999; Robin et al., 1991).

4. STRIVING FOR MATERNAL JUSTICE

Mothers of multiples were concerned that they treat their twins and triplets equally and fairly. It was important not to favor one of the twins or higher-order multiples. There was a need to be fair and equal in the attention given to the multiples. One mother in Anderson and Anderson's (1990) study illustrated how she equalized attention:

> "You think that maybe you're looking at and seeing all the good qualities of one not necessarily to detriment of the other but you just figure you're looking at one more than the other. You say, 'Oh, he's got such lovely blue eyes,' and immediately you think, 'Oh, he's [the other twin] got lovely blue eyes, too,'—they're just different" (p. 375).

In Robin and colleagues (1988) study the mothers expressed that due to their difficulty to respond immediately to their infants feeding demands and need for attention, each infant needed to be treated on an equal basis with regard to the lack of availability of their mother. The women felt obligated to "*do the same thing*" for each infant (p. 154). Robin and associates termed this the need for equalitarianism. In the Robin et al. (1988) study, mothers used two equalitarian strategies. Some women did everything at the same time for the multiples while other mothers did one activity with one infant and then did the same activity with the other one(s). An example of how one mother treated her infants equally, as a unit, was her use of the same spoon, cup, and plate during feeding times (Goshen-Gottstein, 1980). However, treating the infants as one unit was problematic because it meant that the mothers were insensitive at times to the individual scheduling of each infant. For example, one infant might have to be awakened so that he or she could be fed at the same time time as the others. An example of the second type of equalitarian strategy was demonstrated by a mother in Robin et al.'s (1988) study. During mealtimes, the mother made an effort not to start with the same baby each time. Every morning she would reverse the order of which infant was fed first.

Copyright © 2006. Lippincott Williams & Wilkins. *Study Guide to Accompany Essentials of Nursing Research*, by Denise F. Polit and Cheryl Tatano Beck.

Concerns about maternal justice and equalitarianism remained important for mothers throughout the first year of life of their multiples. Anderson and Anderson (1990) reported that maternal guilt over fairness tended to lessen as the infants grew to approximately 8 months of age; they became more independent, took turns for their mother's attention, and received attention from the twinship itself. All these factors helped to alleviate several of the mothers' guilt over fairness.

Mothers were also concerned that they might give preferential treatment to one of the infants over the others. The mothers expressed that they "*can't have a favorite*" and "*can't be biased*" (Holditch-Davis et al., 1999, p. 207).

5. ACKNOWLEDGING INDIVIDUALITY

The task of individuation referred to the mother's ability to adapt to the differences and needs of each of her multiple infants (Anderson & Anderson, 1990). Mothers expressed their need to distinguish between their multiples and to develop individual styles of relating to their infants. A mother tried to capture the challenge of acknowledging individuality by describing this role as one of being a "*quick change artist*." Often she needed to respond to the playfulness of one of her twins while the other one was crying. "*These are constant changes of mood, back and forth, and a mother needs to put on a different mask for each twin*" (Anderson & Anderson, p. 375).

Mothers' differences in how they related to each of their infants were apparent in the manner in which they spoke to and about them, and how they behaved toward them (Goshen-Gottstein, 1980). Mothers varied in the degree to which they individualized their multiple infants.

Anderson and Anderson (1990) discovered that mothers used the strategies of polarization and differentiation to determine the differences between multiples and to help in the task of individuation. Holditch-Davis and colleagues (1999) also reported a recurring theme from their study was that mothers needed to individualize their multiple infants. Mothers continually compared and contrasted their babies' physical characteristics and personalities. Mothers often polarized their infants by describing them as opposites. However, problems were experienced with attempts of differentiation. Robin et al. (1988) found in their study that mothers had to balance a need for early individualization of their multiples with their wish to merge the infants into a single unit.

■ Summary and Conclusion

This meta-synthesis provides maternal-child nurses with a broader, more inclusive perspective from which to practice that could not have been seen in assessing these six studies individually. For example, in all of the studies the mothers need for treating each infant as an individual was reported; however, in only a few studies was the complicating concern of maternal justice revealed. Mothers striving for equality with their multiples is different than their striving for individualization. Clinicians need to be aware that mothers of multiples are simultaneously grappling with both these concerns as they bear the practical burden of providing child care. While women are still pregnant with their

Copyright © 2006. Lippincott Williams & Wilkins. *Study Guide to Accompany Essentials of Nursing Research*, by Denise F. Polit and Cheryl Tatano Beck.

multiples, nurses can provide anticipatory guidance regarding these guilt-producing issues. It can be extremely helpful to place a pregnant woman in touch with a mother who has already delivered multiples to provide practical, concrete strategies for surviving her first year of child care.

This meta-synthesis does have several limitations that should be noted. The qualitative studies that were located and included in this analysis do not represent all possible responses to mothering multiples. Also, the results do not reflect all variations due to culture or other differences in context. In order to extend these findings, in future studies researchers can address mothering multiples in different cultures (e.g., Hispanic mothers) and with differing demographic characteristics (e.g., single vs. married women).

Cheryl Tatano Beck is a Professor of Nursing, University of Connecticut, School of Nursing, Storrs, CT. She can be reached c/o University of Connecticut, School of Nursing U-26, 231 Glenbrook Road, Storrs, CT 06269-2026 (e-mail: cheryl.beck@uconn.edu).

REFERENCES

Anderson, A., & Anderson, B. (1990). Toward a substantive theory of mother-twin attachment. *MCN, The American Journal of Maternal Child Nursing, 15,* 373–377.

Beck, C. T. (1996). Postpartum depressed mothers' experiences interacting with their children. *Nursing Research, 45,* 98–104.

Barroso, J., & Powell-Cope, G. M. (2000). Meta-synthesis of qualitative research on living with HIV infection. *Qualitative Health Research, 10,* 340–353.

Finfgeld, D. L. (1999) Courage as a process of pushing beyond the struggle. *Qualitative Health Research, 9,* 803–814.

Garel, M., & Blondel, B. (1992). Assessment at 1 year of the psychological consequences of having triplets. *Human Reproduction, 7,* 729–732.

Goshen-Gottstein, E. R. (1980). The mothering of twins, triplets, and quadruplets. *Psychiatry, 43,* 189–204.

Holditch-Davis, D., Roberts, D., & Sandelowski, M. (1999). Early parental interactions with and perceptions of multiple birth infants. *Journal of Advanced Nursing, 30,* 200–210.

Jacobson, G. (1994). The meaning of stressful life experiences in nine-to-eleven-year-old children: A phenomenological study. *Nursing Research, 43,* 95–99.

Jensen, L. A., & Allen, M. N. (1994). A synthesis of qualitative research on wellness-illness. *Qualitative Health Research, 4,* 349–369.

Jensen, L. A., & Allen, M. N. (1996). Meta-synthesis of qualitative findings. *Qualitative Health Research, 6,* 553–560.

Morse, J. M. (1997). Responding to threats to integrity of self. *Advances in Nursing Science, 19,* 21–36.

Noblit, G. W., & Hare, R. D. (1988). *Meta-ethnography: Synthesizing qualitative studies.* Newbury Park, CA: Sage.

Robin, M., Bydlowski, M., Cahen, F., & Josse, D. (1991). Maternal reactions to the birth of triplets. *Acta Genet Med Gemellol, 40,* 41–51.

Robin, M., Josse, D., & Tourrette, C. (1988). Mother/twin interaction during early childhood. *Acta Genet Med Gemellol, 37,* 151–159.

Sandelowski, M. (1997). "To Be of Use": Enhance the utility of qualitative research. *Nursing Outlook, 45,* 125–132.

Sandelowski, M., Docherty, S., & Emden, C. (1997). Qualitative meta-synthesis: Issues and techniques. *Research in Nursing and Health, 20,* 365–371.

Schreiber, R., Crooks, D., & Stern, P. N. (1997). Qualitative meta-analysis. In J. M. Morse (Ed.), *Completing a qualitative project* (pp. 311–326). Thousand Oaks, CA Sage.

Wismont, J. M. (2000). The lived pregnancy experience of women in prison. *Journal of Midwifery and Women's Health, 45,* 292–300.

Copyright © 2006. Lippincott Williams & Wilkins. *Study Guide to Accompany Essentials of Nursing Research,* by Denise F. Polit and Cheryl Tatano Beck.

ANSWER KEY

■ Chapter 1

A. Matching exercises

1. a   2. b   3. d   4. b   5. a   6. b   7. d   8. b   9. c   10. a

B. Completion exercises
1. Florence Nightingale
2. Nursing education
3. National Institute of Nursing Research
4. Clinical practice
5. Tradition
6. Naturalistic
7. Positivism
8. Empirical
9. Determinism
10. Generalizability
11. Reductionist
12. Quantitative research
13. Qualitative research
14. Identification

C.1. For crossword puzzle answers, see page 322.

A.1.
1. a   2. c   3. b   4. a   5. c   6. a   7. c
8. c   9. c   10. b   11. a   12. a   13. b   14. b   15. c

■ Chapter 2

A. Matching exercises

A.2.
1. b   2. c   3. a   4. d   5. c   6. c   7. b   8. d

B. Completion exercises

1. Subjects, study participants
2. Concepts
3. Variable
4. Independent
5. Dependent, outcome
6. Independent
7. Extraneous
8. Data
9. Operational definitions
10. Qualitative

Copyright © 2006. Lippincott Williams & Wilkins. *Study Guide to Accompany Essentials of Nursing Research*, by Denise F. Polit and Cheryl Tatano Beck.

11. Patterns of association
12. Cause-and-effect (causal)
13. Inductive
14. Deductive

15. Reliability, validity
16. Trustworthiness
17. Triangulation
18. Generalizability, transferability

C.1. For crossword puzzle answers, see page 322.

■ Chapter 3

A. Matching exercises

A.1.
1. a   2. b   3. a   4. c   5. a
6. c   7. d   8. c   9. b   10. a

A.2.
1. c   2. b   3. a   4. a   5. b
6. d   7. e   8. b   9. c   10. d

B. Completion Exercises
1. Intervention (treatment)
2. Grounded theory, phenomenology, ethnography
3. Phenomenology
4. Grounded theory
5. Quantitative
6. Hypotheses
7. Clinical fieldwork
8. Research design
9. Population
10. Sample
11. Data analysis
12. Pilot study
13. Research report
14. Dissemination
15. Gaining entrée
16. Gatekeepers
17. Emergent
18. Saturation

C.1. For crossword puzzle answers, see page 322.

■ Chapter 4

A. Matching exercises

1. c   2. d   3. b   4. a   5. c   6. e
7. d   8. b   9. c   10. e   11. b   12. d

B. Completion exercises
1. Oral report, poster session
2. Journal articles
3. Abstract
4. Headings
5. Introduction
6. Methods
7. Statistical test
8. Level of significance
9. Themes (categories)
10. Results

C.1. For crossword puzzle answers, see page 323.

Copyright © 2006. Lippincott Williams & Wilkins. *Study Guide to Accompany Essentials of Nursing Research*, by Denise F. Polit and Cheryl Tatano Beck.

■ Chapter 5

A. Matching exercises

1. d   2. b   3. c   4. b   5. a   6. d
7. b   8. a   9. c   10. a   11. b   12. d

B. Completion exercises
1. Dilemmas
2. Nuremberg code
3. *Belmont Report*
4. Harm
5. Minimal risks
6. Self-determination
7. Full disclosure
8. Anonymity
9. Vulnerable
10. Institutional Review Boards
11. Informed consent
12. Fabrication, falsification, plagiarism

C.1. For crossword puzzle answers, see page 323.

■ Chapter 6

A. Matching exercises

A.1.
1. b   2. c   3. a   4. b   5. a   6. c   7. b   8. a

A.2.
1. a   2. c   3. d   4. a   5. b   6. d   7. a   8. c

9. b   10. d   11. b   12. c   13. b   14. a   15. c

B. Completion exercises
1. Research problem
2. Research question
3. Research aims, objectives
4. Experience, literature, social issues, theory, external sources
5. Qualitative
6. Introduction
7. Verbs
8. Relationship
9. Two
10. Independent, dependent
11. Complex
12. Null (statistical)

C.1. For crossword puzzle answers, see page 323.

■ Chapter 7

A. Matching exercises

1. a   2. b   3. d   4. e   5. c   6. a   7. e   8. d   9. e   10. b

B. Completion exercises

Copyright © 2006. Lippincott Williams & Wilkins. *Study Guide to Accompany Essentials of Nursing Research,* by Denise F. Polit and Cheryl Tatano Beck.

1. Research problems (ideas)
2. Research findings (results)
3. Primary
4. CINAHL
5. Subject

6. Textword
7. Quotes
8. Gaps
9. Critical summary
10. Tentativeness

C.1. For crossword puzzle answers, see page 324.

■ Chapter 8

A. Matching exercises

A.1. 1. c   2. e   3. d   4. e   5. d   6. a   7. b   8. d

A.2. 1. c   2. d   3. g   4. a   5. f   6. b   7. h   8. e

B. Completion exercises
1. Invented (created, constructed)
2. Hypotheses
3. Framework
4. Conceptual models
5. Words

6. Person, environment, health, nursing
7. Induction
8. Health Promotion Model
9. Borrowed theories, shared theories
10. Grounded

C.1. For crossword puzzle answers, see page 324.

■ Chapter 9

A. Matching exercises

1. b   2. b   3. a   4. d   5. b

6. a   7. d   8. a   9. b   10. d

B. Completion exercises

1. Comparison
2. Independent
3. Treatment (intervention)
4. Systematic bias
5. Random assignment
6. Pretest (baseline measure)
7. Factorial design
8. Levels
9. Double-blind
10. Crossover (repeated measure)
11. Causality (causal relationships)
12. Comparison

13. Preexperimental
14. Time series
15. Equal (equivalent)
16. Nonexperimental
17. Correlational
18. Independent
19. Causation
20. Retrospective
21. Case-control
22. Longitudinal
23. Follow-up studies
24. Constancy

Copyright © 2006. Lippincott Williams & Wilkins. *Study Guide to Accompany Essentials of Nursing Research*, by Denise F. Polit and Cheryl Tatano Beck.

25. Protocols
26. Generalizability
27. Internal
28. Selection

29. Maturation
30. History
31. External
32. Statistical conclusion

C.1. For crossword puzzle answers, see page 324.

■ Chapter 10

A. Matching exercises

1. b   2. a   3. d   4. c   5. b

6. a   7. b   8. c   9. d   10. c

B. Completion exercises
1. Emergent
2. Bricoleurs
3. Anthropology, psychology, sociology
4. Cultures
5. Macroethnography, microethnography
6. Researcher as instrument
7. Essence
8. Spatiality, corporeality, temporality, relationality

9. Reflexive
10. Hermeneutics
11. Grounded theory
12. Constant comparison
13. Formal grounded theory
14. Historical research
15. Critical theory
16. Participatory action research

C.1. For crossword puzzle answers, see page 325.

■ Chapter 11

A. Matching exercises

1. a, b, c, e   2. b   3. e   4. d   5. c

6. a   7. b   8. a, b, c, d, e, f   9. a   10. f

B. Completion exercises
1. Randomized clinical trials (RCTs)
2. Pilot test
3. Process (implementation)
4. Net
5. Cost-benefit
6. Outcomes research
7. Methods

8. Telephone
9. Unit of analysis
10. Case study
11. Complementary
12. Validity
13. Instruments
14. Black box

C.1. For crossword puzzle answers, see page 325.

Copyright © 2006. Lippincott Williams & Wilkins. *Study Guide to Accompany Essentials of Nursing Research*, by Denise F. Polit and Cheryl Tatano Beck.

■ Chapter 12

A. Matching exercises

A.1.
1. c	2. a	3. d	4. b	5. d
6. b	7. c	8. d	9. a	10. d

A.2.
1. b	2. c	3. a	4. b	5. b
6. c	7. a	8. a	9. d	10. b

B. Completion exercises
1. Sample
2. Representativeness
3. Biased
4. Homogeneous
5. Judgmental (or purposeful)
6. Strata
7. Accidental; volunteer
8. Simple random
9. Sampling frame
10. Weighting
11. Multistage
12. Sampling interval
13. Sampling error
14. Accessible
15. Increases
16. 30
17. Information
18. Homogeneous; maximum variation
19. Typical case
20. Theoretical
21. Confirming, disconfirming
22. Key informants

C.1. For crossword puzzle answers, see page 325.

■ Chapter 13

A. Matching exercises

A.1.
1. a, c	2. a, b	3. b, c	4. c	5. b
6. b	7. a, b, c	8. a, b	9. a, b, c	10. a, b

A.2.
1. b	2. a	3. c	4. a	5. d	6. a
7. a	8. b	9. d	10. c	11. c	12. b

B. Completion exercises
1. Structure, quantifiability, researcher obtrusiveness, objectivity
2. Researcher obtrusiveness
3. Biophysiologic
4. Inexpensive
5. Self-reports
6. Grand tour
7. Topic guide
8. Focus group interview
9. Critical incidents
10. Think-aloud
11. Closed-ended (fixed-alternative)
12. Dichotomous
13. Declarative

Copyright © 2006. Lippincott Williams & Wilkins. *Study Guide to Accompany Essentials of Nursing Research*, by Denise F. Polit and Cheryl Tatano Beck.

14. Reversed
15. Semantic differential
16. Visual analog scale (VAS)
17. Extreme response set
18. 9, 11
19. Vignettes
20. Behavior
21. Reactivity

22. Participant observation
23. Log (field diary)
24. Category system
25. Time sampling
26. Trained
27. In vivo
28. In vitro

C.1. For crossword puzzle answers, see page 326.

■ Chapter 14

A. Matching exercises

A.1.
1. a   2. c   3. d   4. c   5. b
6. d   7. b   8. a   9. c   10. d

A.2.
1. a   2. c   3. b   4. d   5. a   6. b

B. Completion exercises
1. Attributes (characteristics)
2. Quantification
3. Rules
4. True score
5. Measurement error
6. True score
7. Stability
8. Coefficient alpha (Cronbach's alpha)
9. Interrater (interobserver) reliability
10. Valid
11. Face
12. Content

13. Predictive
14. Construct
15. Psychometric assessment
16. Sensitivity, specificity
17. Credibility, dependability, confirmability, transferability
18. Prolonged engagement
19. Data source triangulation
20. Member checking
21. Confirmability
22. Inquiry audit

C.1. For crossword puzzle answers, see page 326.

■ Chapter 15

A. Matching exercises

A.1.
1. d   2. a   3. d   4. b   5. c   6. a
7. b   8. d   9. c   10. b   11. b   12. a

Copyright © 2006. Lippincott Williams & Wilkins. *Study Guide to Accompany Essentials of Nursing Research,* by Denise F. Polit and Cheryl Tatano Beck.

A.2.

1. b	2. a	3. c	4. d	5. b
6. b	7. a	8. a	9. c	10. a

A.3.

1. b	2. a	3. d	4. b	5. c
6. a	7. a	8. a	9. d	10. a

B. Completion exercises

1. Classification (categorization)
2. Ordinal
3. Zero
4. Equal distances
5. Parameter
6. Frequency distribution
7. Frequency polygons
8. Symmetric
9. Negatively
10. Unimodal
11. Normal distribution (bell-shaped curve)
12. Central tendency
13. Variability
14. Homogeneous
15. Standard deviation
16. Bivariate statistics
17. Negative (inverse)
18. Pearson's r (product–moment correlation coefficient)
19. Inferential statistics
20. Normal
21. Type I
22. Parametric
23. Levels of significance
24. Type II
25. t-test, analysis of variance
26. F-ratio
27. Chi-squared test (χ^2 test)
28. Multiple regression
29. R
30. .00, 1.00
31. Analysis of covariance
32. Covariate
33. Factor analysis
34. Discriminant function analysis, logistic regression
35. Logistic regression
36. Path analysis, LISREL

C.1. For crossword puzzle answers, see page 326.

■ Chapter 16

A. Matching exercises

1. a, b, c	2. a	3. b	4. a, b, c	5. a
6. c	7. b	8. c	9. a, b	10. d

B. Completion exercises

1. Simultaneously
2. Comprehending, synthesizing, theorizing, recontextualizing
3. Indexing, categorizing
4. Conceptual file
5. Computerized methods
6. Themes or patterns
7. Quasi-statistics
8. Domain, taxonomic, componential, theme
9. Phenomenological
10. Detailed
11. Constitutive pattern
12. Paradigm cases

Copyright © 2006. Lippincott Williams & Wilkins. *Study Guide to Accompany Essentials of Nursing Research*, by Denise F. Polit and Cheryl Tatano Beck.

13. Constant comparison
14. Open coding

15. Selective
16. Basic social process

C.1. For crossword puzzle answers, see page 327.

■ Chapter 17

A. Matching exercises

A.1.
| 1. b | 2. c | 3. b | 4. d | 5. b |
| 6. a | 7. d | 8. c | 9. a | 10. a |

A.2.
| 1. b | 2. c | 3. d | 4. b | 5. b |
| 6. a | 7. c | 8. d | | |

B. Completion exercises
1. Accuracy (credibility)
2. Hypotheses
3. Causation
4. Their data
5. Important (useful)
6. Decisions

7. Strengths, weaknesses (virtues, flaws)
8. Substantive/theoretical
9. Methodologic
10. Ethical
11. Interpretive
12. Stylistic/presentational

C.1. For crossword puzzle answers, see page 327.

■ Chapter 18

A. Matching exercises

| 1. c | 2. d | 3. a | 4. b |
| 5. d | 6. a | 7. a | 8. b |

B. Completion exercises
1. Instrumental (direct) utilization
2. Gap
3. Conduct and Utilization of Research in Nursing (CURN)
4. Research utilization, evidence-based practice
5. Cochrane
6. Evidence hierarchy

7. Meta-analyses of RCTs
8. Stetler
9. Knowledge-focused, problem-focused
10. Integrative review
11. Implementation potential
12. Ancestry, descendancy
13. Sensitivity
14. Noblit and Hare

C.1. For crossword puzzle answers, see page 327.

Copyright © 2006. Lippincott Williams & Wilkins. *Study Guide to Accompany Essentials of Nursing Research*, by Denise F. Polit and Cheryl Tatano Beck.

Puzzle 1:

```
E V I D E N C E - B A S E D
M                       E B M
P A R A D I G M     N A T
I   E   E       H       E     E
I   P O S I T I V I S M   R   X
I   L   C       E   E   M     P
C   I   R N C N R T R I A L
A   C   I       A   H   N     A
    A P P L   Q   R       I   N
    T   T O U T C O M E S
R   I   I   A   H       M     T
I   O   O   L   Y   U         I
N   N I N R   I       T N     O
A     N       T R A D I T I O N
H I S T O R Y         L   H
```

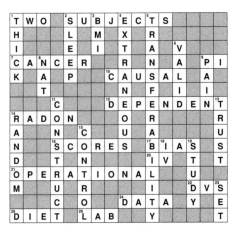

```
T W O   S U B J E C T S
H       L   M   X   R
I       E   I   T   A   V
C A N C E R     R   N A   P I
K   A   P   C A U S A L   A
    T       N   F   I     I
      C   D E P E N D E N T
R A D O N   O   R         R
A     N   C U   A         U
    S C O R E S B I A S   S
    T   N     I V   T     T
O P E R A T I O N A L   U
M   U   R     I     D V   S
    C   O   D A T A   Y   E
D I E T   L A B     Y     T
```

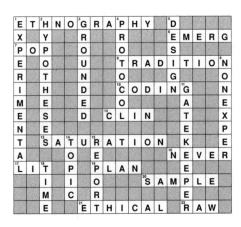

```
E T H N O G R A P H Y   D
X   Y   R     R       E M E R G
P O P   O     O       S
E   O   U   T R A D I T I O   N
R   T   N   O       G     O   O
I   H   D   C O D I N G   N   N
M   E   E   O         A   E   E
E   S   D C L I N     T       X
N   E     L         E         P
T   S A T U R A T I O N   K   E
A     O   E       N E V E R   E
L I T   P P L A N     E
    I   I O     S A M P L E
    M   C R           E
    E   E T H I C A L   R A W
```

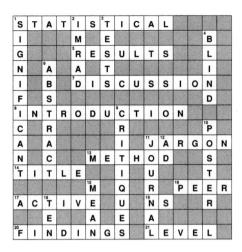

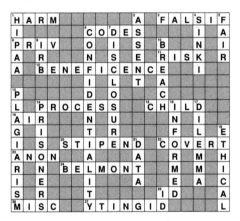

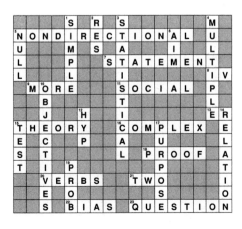

Copyright © 2006. Lippincott Williams & Wilkins. *Study Guide to Accompany Essentials of Nursing Research,* by Denise F. Polit and Cheryl Tatano Beck.

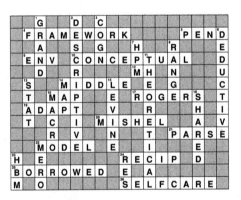

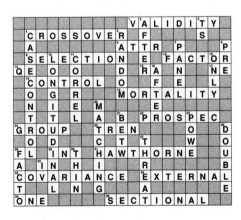

Copyright © 2006. Lippincott Williams & Wilkins. *Study Guide to Accompany Essentials of Nursing Research*, by Denise F. Polit and Cheryl Tatano Beck.

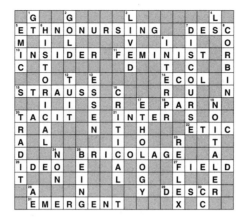

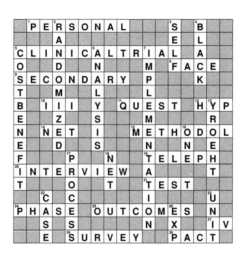

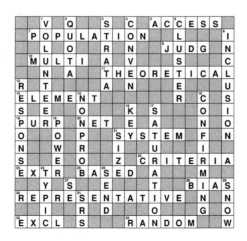

Copyright © 2006. Lippincott Williams & Wilkins. *Study Guide to Accompany Essentials of Nursing Research*, by Denise F. Polit and Cheryl Tatano Beck.

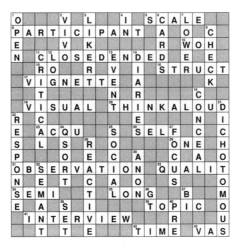

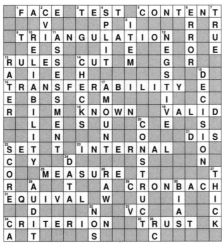

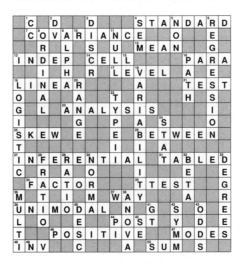

Copyright © 2006. Lippincott Williams & Wilkins. *Study Guide to Accompany Essentials of Nursing Research*, by Denise F. Polit and Cheryl Tatano Beck.

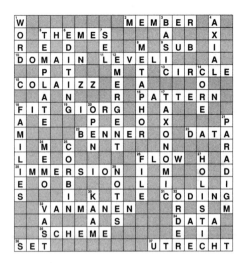

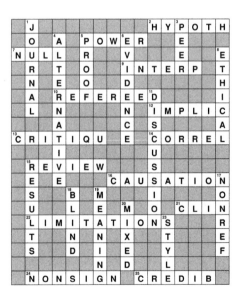

Copyright © 2006. Lippincott Williams & Wilkins. *Study Guide to Accompany Essentials of Nursing Research*, by Denise F. Polit and Cheryl Tatano Beck.